THE SUFFERING STRANGER

THE SUFFERING STRANGER

Hermeneutics for Everyday
Clinical Practice

Donna M. Orange

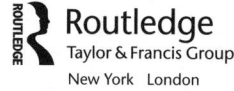
Routledge
Taylor & Francis Group
New York London

Routledge
Taylor & Francis Group
711 Third Avenue
New York, NY 10017

Routledge
Taylor & Francis Group
27 Church Road
Hove, East Sussex BN3 2FA

© 2011 by Taylor and Francis Group, LLC
Routledge is an imprint of Taylor & Francis Group, an Informa business

Printed in the United States of America on acid-free paper
10 9 8 7 6 5 4 3 2

International Standard Book Number: 978-0-415-87403-8 (Hardback) 978-0-415-87404-5 (Paperback)

For permission to photocopy or use material electronically from this work, please access www.copyright.com (http://www.copyright.com/) or contact the Copyright Clearance Center, Inc. (CCC), 222 Rosewood Drive, Danvers, MA 01923, 978-750-8400. CCC is a not-for-profit organization that provides licenses and registration for a variety of users. For organizations that have been granted a photocopy license by the CCC, a separate system of payment has been arranged.

Trademark Notice: Product or corporate names may be trademarks or registered trademarks, and are used only for identification and explanation without intent to infringe.

Library of Congress Cataloging-in-Publication Data

Orange, Donna M., 1944- author.
   The suffering stranger : hermeneutics for everyday clinical practice / Donna M. Orange.
      p. ; cm.
   Includes bibliographical references.
   ISBN 978-0-415-87403-8 (hardcover : alk. paper) -- ISBN 978-0-415-87404-5 (softcover : alk. paper) -- ISBN 978-0-203-86363-3 (e-book)
   1. Psychoanalysis--Philosophy. 2. Hermeneutics. I. Title.
   [DNLM: 1. Psychoanalytic Theory. 2. Humanism. 3. Philosophy. 4. Psychoanalysis--history. WM 460]

BF175.4.P45O753 2011
150.19'5--dc22
                                                                                             2010046619

Visit the Taylor & Francis Web site at
http://www.taylorandfrancis.com

and the Routledge Web site at
http://www.routledgementalhealth.com

> Remember only
> That I was innocent and, just like
> you, mortal on that day,
> I too, had a face marked by rage, by pity and joy,
> Quite simply, a human face!
>
> —**Benjamin Fontane,** *Exodus*

To my patients,
and
to my sisters and brothers

Contents

Preface		ix
Chapter 1	What Is Hermeneutics?	1
Chapter 2	The Suffering Stranger and the Hermeneutics of Trust	37
Chapter 3	Sándor Ferenczi: The Analyst of Last Resort and the Hermeneutics of Trauma	73
Chapter 4	Frieda Fromm-Reichmann: Incommunicable Loneliness	111
Chapter 5	D. W. Winnicott: Humanitarian Without Sentimentality	137
Chapter 6	Heinz Kohut: Glimpsing the Hidden Suffering	175
Chapter 7	Bernard Brandchaft: Liberating the Incarcerated Spirit	205
Afterword: The Next Step		237
References		239
Index		259

Preface

My last book, *Thinking for Clinicians*, attempted to bring philosophers into conversation with psychoanalysts and with other humanistically oriented psychotherapists. Now I attempt the project in reverse: to present a group of my favorite subversives in the history of psychoanalysis and to bring them into conversation with Gadamerian hermeneutics and Lévinasian ethics. None of these five extraordinary clinicians—Sándor Ferenczi, Frieda Fromm-Reichmann, Donald Winnicott, Heinz Kohut, and Bernard Brandchaft—*intended* to subvert the official program of psychoanalysis, but, faithful to what they were learning from their patients, they became subversives in spite of their best efforts to remain respectful to Freud especially and to remain within the communities that had nurtured them. Their common devotion to the needs of the suffering patient allowed them to question doctrine, dogma, and traditional practice. Thus, for me, they seem kindred spirits to each other.

On the philosophical end, Hans-Georg Gadamer and Emmanuel Lévinas will be familiar to readers of my previous excursion, but I will reintroduce them here, in their specific relevance for this dialogue. My students and colleagues have long extracted promises from me to write a book on hermeneutics (the theory and practice of interpretation); I hereby repay that debt, while sneaking in what has become a further passion: to understand as fully as I can the ethical and vocational aspects of our profession.

From its earliest years, psychoanalysis has included a strand, often hidden, often quite violently silenced, that offered an alternative to its rationalistic, "investigative," "scientific," and more detached and establishment-protecting elements. This voice, the therapeutic counterpoint, often condemned as the *furor sanandi* (passion to heal), became buried under contempt and shame as few found courage to write of their convictions and experiences. The more maternal voices, like Ferenczi, Kohut, and Winnicott, have all faced speculation about their sexuality. Biography apart, they were plainly not tough enough to confront the tradition or their patients—so the story goes, no matter the textual evidence—as we will see later. Many therapists, dissatisfied with psychoanalysis on various grounds, simply found their way into other forms of psychotherapy, though we may now be slowly finding each other again in our common therapeutic project. Unfortunately, psychoanalysis, even in many contemporary forms, has remained a project for the tough-minded, for those who predominantly practice what we will be calling the hermeneutics of suspicion. This book intends to suggest—to psychoanalysts and other psychotherapists—that we can do our work in another spirit, without relegating our more compassionate hermeneuts to the contempt file where they have been too often placed.

The first chapters concern hermeneutics and Lévinasian ethics, followed by five on Sándor Ferenczi, Frieda Fromm-Reichmann, Donald Woods Winnicott, Heinz Kohut, and Bernard Brandchaft.* Recognizing that context generates our hermeneutics (Atwood & Stolorow, 1993) to a very great extent, I begin these five chapters with short introductions to the life and work of the thinker and

---

* Other candidates, reluctantly passed over for reasons of time, included Ian Suttie, Emmanuel Ghent, and Hans Loewald. I did not consider for this book people who are still working and might have refuted my account of their attitudes!

follow with considerations of the central hermeneutic (interpretive) approach of each. This book does not contain a summary of the important ideas of each thinker, as these are easily available elsewhere, and some are quite familiar to most readers. Nor have I tried to defend these groundbreakers from their critics, or even to avoid selective readings and consider the full complexity of their ideas, as these tasks would have distracted from my purposes. Instead, I want to engage these innovative psychoanalysts precisely as interpreters and as those who have seen the face of the other and heard the voice of the stranger in the ethical sense. If I have quoted them extensively, my purpose has been to let their unique voices, too often silenced, speak out.*

The task of thanking those whose generosity and support have made this book possible for me to write daunts me, not only because I am bound to overlook and injure someone but also because it seems really irreverent to begin or end. Once again my own psychoanalytic communities, Institute for the Psychoanalytic Study of Subjectivity (IPSS, New York) and Istituto di Specializzazione in Psicologia Psicoanalitica del Se' e Psicoanalisi Relazionale (ISIPSe', Roma, Milano), as well as my study groups and workshops around the world, are unobtrusive but important, generative, and sustaining contexts. Some to whom I feel deep gratitude I have never met or scarcely know, but they have made the work of Ferenczi available and spoken for him to many of us, in particular Andre Haynal, Judith Dupont, Judith Vida, Emmanuel Berman, and others too numerous to mention. Others—Susanna Federici-Nebbiosi, Kathleen Fischer, Manfred Frank, Thomas Hart, Chris Jaenicke, Elizabeth Liebert, Gianni Nebbiosi, Frank Staemmler, Veronique Zanetti—share with me a bond of friendship that supports the risks this book involves. More immediately, thank you to my chapter readers: George Atwood, Elizabeth Corpt, Shelley Doctors, Peter Kravitz, Hilary Maddux, Michael Reison, and Robert Stolorow, whose suggestions made the book much better

---

* Emphasis in all quoted text is from the original, unless otherwise noted.

and saved me from embarrassing errors. All provided needed moral support as well. My very dear friend, Lynne Jacobs, and my husband, Donald Braue, have both read everything at least once and have been with me in countless ways through the whole project. Of course errors remain, and these, as well as all the opinions, belong to me. Kristopher Spring of Routledge has warmly supported this book; without his enthusiasm I might not have persevered. To go back to the beginning, George Atwood has inspired my work in the direction this book has taken from the time we met in 1987 and has been my teacher, friend, and dialogic interlocutor, even when we disagree. Bob Stolorow, fellow philosopher, has always believed in me. To come to the moment if not to the end, Don has trusted that this book could be important and has allowed it to take over our lives for months as if I were the suffering stranger to whom he has been responding. Without being a therapist, he embodies everything this book tries to describe, and no words of mine suffice to thank him.

1
What Is Hermeneutics?

> *The person who is understanding does not know and judge as one who stands apart and unaffected but rather he thinks along with the other from the perspective of a specific bond of belonging, as if he too were affected.*
>
> —**Gadamer**

Hermeneutics? It may seem strange for someone as allergic to jargon as my students know me to be to embark on a book about an experience-distant term like *hermeneutics*. Still, I plead for its admission to our conversation on the grounds that it will help us tremendously to understand what we do as clinicians and to discern the different spirits in which we may approach what we do. So let us begin to approach the word itself.*

Hermeneutics, the study of interpretation, historically functioned as an adjunct discipline, first to theology and later to history, literature, and jurisprudence. Richard Palmer (2002), historian of hermeneutics, wrote a genial history of the origins of the word:

> Hermes, you will recall from the *Iliad* and the *Odyssey*, was the messenger of the gods. He carried messages from Zeus to everybody else, especially from the divine realm and level down to the human level. In doing so, he had to bridge an ontological gap, a gap

---

* The substantive form is either *hermeneutics* or *hermeneutic*, and I use both. The adjective is *hermeneutic*. To indicate the practitioner of this art, I use *hermeneut* in preference to *hermeneuticist*, which I find awkward and ugly.

> between the thinking of the gods and that of humans. According to legend, he had (1) a mysterious helmet which could make him invisible and then suddenly reappear, (2) magical wings on his sandals to carry him swiftly over long distances, and (3) a magical wand that could put you to sleep or wake you up. So he not only bridged physical distances and the ontological gap between divine and human being, he bridged the difference between the visible and the invisible, and between dreams and waking, between the unconscious and the conscious. He is the quicksilver god ["Mercury" in Latin] of sudden insights, ideas, inspirations. And he is also the trickster god of thefts, highway robbery, and of sudden windfalls of good luck. Norman O. Brown wrote a book about him titled *Hermes the Thief*. Hermes is the god of crossroads and boundaries, where piles of rocks (Herms) were placed to honor him. As psychopomp, Hermes led the dead into the underworld, so he "crossed the line" between the living and the dead, between the living human world and the underworld of Hades. Hermes is truly the "god of the gaps," of the margins, the boundaries, the *limins* of many things. (p. 2)

Originally the study of methods for interpreting sacred texts, hermeneutics served theological purposes. From the time of the early 19th-century romantics, it broadened its scope to include history, aesthetics, and whatever belonged to the humanities and social sciences generally. Given Freud's emphasis on interpretation, it might have seemed obvious that psychoanalysis would have been seen as a hermeneutic study.* Unfortunately, because of his even stronger insistence on the status of psychoanalysis as natural science, our awareness of psychoanalysis as hermeneutics has arrived only more recently, and with some reasonable cautions (Friedman, 2000; Steiner, 1995). Furthermore, other psychotherapeutic traditions, needing to distance themselves from what they have understood—with considerable justification—as an excessively intellectualized interpretive therapeutics in psychoanalysis, have also missed out on what a hermeneutic sensibility can offer.†

---

* See Sass (1989) for a discussion of the complex relations between psychoanalysis, humanistic views, and the history of hermeneutics.
† Gestalt therapists learned, for example, to "never, never interpret," but now one of their prominent theorists (Staemmler, 2007, 2009) makes extensive use of Gadamer's dialogic hermeneutics.

In the hands of phenomenologists, first Martin Heidegger but principally Hans-Georg Gadamer, hermeneutics became a general philosophy of dialogical understanding, serving philosophy, the social sciences, and beyond. Now, I suggest, dialogical hermeneutics can become the partner of an ethical clinical sensibility and sense of vocation best expressed in the ethical phenomenology of Emmanuel Lévinas, in whose thinking each of us bears an infinite responsibility to the face of the suffering stranger.

This book therefore has a double task: (a) to explain and illustrate the richness of a hermeneutic clinical sensibility and (b) to illustrate that such a sensibility responds well to the ethical imperative of hospitality to the suffering stranger that we find described in the challenging writings of Emmanuel Lévinas.

This project thus approaches hermeneutics in three ways: (a) it attempts to trace the history of hermeneutics in a user-friendly way so that humanistic psychotherapists of all traditions can recognize their work as hermeneutic and make use of the resources that philosophical hermeneutics offers, (b) it studies work of several especially humanistic psychoanalysts—because this is my own tradition—to show both how these clinicians developed a hermeneutic therapeutics and how a dialogic hermeneutics understands both persons and texts, and (c) it links a dialogic clinical hermeneutics to an ethical concern, shared by these clinicians and by the philosophers Hans-Georg Gadamer and Emmanuel Lévinas, for the voice and the face of the other.

HISTORY OF HERMENEUTICS: SCHLEIERMACHER

Let us begin with the hermeneutics of the courageous* romantic-era theologian Friedrich Schleiermacher (1768–1834), German theologian and philosopher, contemporary of Goethe and

---

* For my appreciation of Schleiermacher, I am indebted to philosopher and scholar of the early romantics Manfred Frank, who often told me stories of Schleiermacher's personal courage.

Beethoven, an important resource for the so-called hermeneutic turn in contemporary psychoanalysis.

The contemporary or post-Freudian psychoanalysis to which I refer includes British independents and American relationalists, made up, broadly speaking, of interpersonalists, psychoanalytic self psychologists, as well as phenomenologically oriented intersubjectivists and many clinicians worldwide inspired by various relational ideas. We have largely turned away from Freud's natural-science-based psychoanalysis whose "interpretations" explained to the patient* his or her instinct-based complexes and conflicts. The analyst used to be the silent and distant expert authority on the patient's unconscious conflicts over sex and aggression, the archaeologist/excavator of the depths. Now, instead, most of us work dialogically, hoping more to understand suffering via its background in lived intersubjective experience than to explain or translate unconscious "mental" contents. We believe that our groping together for words for whatever we can come to understand becomes a healing and a liberating process. We realize that the analyst's personal history, our own intimate *Selbstvertrautheit* (Frank, 2000),† is involved at every moment in our effort to contact and to understand the suffering other (Orange, 1995) and that the other in turn is always affecting us. Our thinking and our practice has changed profoundly from the distant and impersonal world of what we often call "classical" psychoanalysis.

So what has Schleiermacher to offer us, beyond the example of a man who was willing to place himself at risk for people‡ whom

---

* Throughout this book, as in my other writings, I use the word patient (from the Latin *patior*, "to suffer, to undergo") to refer to the human beings with whom I work. Clients would be people with whom I primarily have business relationships. Patients are fellow sufferers.
† I am using his very carefully defined concept loosely here. He speaks of unmediated familiarity (*Vertrautheit*) and says, "One is conscious of how one feels (or of 'what it is like') even when one does not know in the slightest how one should classify the feeling. (It could happen that I am in love even though I lack a valid theory of love, or even lack the concept itself)" (Frank, 2000, p. 194).
‡ See, for example, his letters on behalf of the emancipation of the Jews in Prussia (Schleiermacher & Schmidt, 2001).

others considered less than fully human? I have chosen three themes: (a) his recognition that understanding is hard, if not impossible, work; (b) what I would call his proto-fallibilism; and (c) his insistence on holism, or what today we might call complexity, an attitude that resists the enticements of reductionism that continue to tempt clinicians.

Schleiermacher taught that understanding, whether of texts or of people, was hard work and always work in progress. Because every child learns a language, and because so much of daily life passes without our noticing misunderstandings, he had to tell us explicitly that "misunderstanding occurs as a matter of course, and so understanding must be willed and sought at every point" (Schleiermacher & Kimmerle, 1977, p. 110). In contrast to what he called the "lax practice" of hermeneutics, which assumes understanding (Schleiermacher & Bowie, 1998), the "rigorous practice" or "strict practice" always required this hardworking attitude. In my clinical experience, patients are often greatly surprised and relieved when I quote this to them; they have expected themselves to understand their spouses and their partners to understand them, and likewise their analysts or therapists. To see that understanding requires hard effort, and that this should be expected, is already a start in hermeneutics. This work requires, Schleiermacher taught, constant attention to both content and feeling tone of whatever we seek to understand. Moreover, this rigorous practice is a no-fault enterprise: "Non-understanding is partly indeterminacy, partly ambiguity of the content. So it is thought of without any fault on the part of the utterer" (Schleiermacher & Bowie, 1998, p. 227). He seems to have believed that if I want to understand I must go toward the utterer, not force the utterer to come to me. Not surprisingly, then, my interest in hermeneutics helps me to work with patients who suffer from dreadful, even suicidal, forms of shame: If everything is just something to understand, not to despise or to blame, my patients' self-hatred sometimes gives way to a more self-forgiving *Selbstvertrautheit* (self-familiarity, sense of being at home with oneself).

Even the psychotherapist's struggles to understand patterns of seemingly intractable misery can become more bearable in light of this "rigorous practice." My patient who seems to have everything, including everything that I have never had, but continues to return to a truly abusive partner, one who throws hot soup on her in anger and rages at her in front of friends and family, confounds me. Then I remember that understanding is a difficult practice and that there is clearly something we have not understood together yet. Yes, Schleiermacher helps.

Indeed, Schleiermacher claimed elsewhere, no one, strictly speaking, can understand another person. What can this mean? Schleiermacher held that the art of hermeneutics had two indispensible elements, the grammatical and the psychological:

> In order to complete the grammatical side of interpretation it would be necessary to have complete knowledge of the language. In order to complete the psychological side it would be necessary to have a complete knowledge of the person. Since in both cases such complete knowledge is impossible, it is necessary to move back and forth between the grammatical and psychological sides, and no rules can stipulate exactly how to do this. (Schleiermacher & Kimmerle, 1977, p. 100)

This brings us to our second theme. He replaced confidence in Cartesian "clear and distinct ideas" with awareness that all our understanding is partial and fallible, that it comes piecemeal and in degrees. It may be that Schleiermacher's famous or infamous method of intuitive understanding embodied this proto-fallibilism. If, perhaps, he meant that the interpreter makes a reasonable guess, taking historical and other forms of context into account, at the meaning of a text, and then tests it out, this would be very similar to the method of hypothesis in Charles Sanders Peirce (1931). Taking a dream as a text, for example, a clinician might ask whether being chased feels like anything in previous or current life, and work from there. One always intends interpretation as tentative and fallible. Schleiermacher even termed his oscillating intersubjective search for truth—in Plato's spirit—*dialectic*.

In clinical work, we work in this spirit hundreds of times a day, testing, discarding, and provisionally keeping our hunches. The famous "squiggle" game of British psychoanalyst D. W. Winnicott (1971), in which both patient and analyst added lines to a drawing until something emerged, was a form of hermeneutic play, I think. Many of us psychoanalysts probably do the same thing with words as we wonder together about symptoms, dreams, daydreams, bits of traumatic memory, and such. Whenever the understanding seems adequate for the moment, or unable to be taken further for the moment, we let it go for the moment. In this way both patient and analyst become fallibilists, less obsessive about being right and certain, less caught in traumatically generated either–or positions (Orange, 2011). Knowing gradually becomes disengaged from the search for certainty and becomes a shared project.

In Schleiermacher's own words, in his explanation of the "psychological" aspects of hermeneutic understanding, we find the following, written at least 130 years before Winnicott's squiggle or before Gadamer's dialogic hermeneutics:

> If we consider a conversation, this is first of all a completely free state, which is based, not on any specific objective intention, but only on the mutually stimulating exchange of thoughts. ... But the conversation does easily get fixed on something and that is even striven for by both sides. In this way a common development of thoughts and a particular relationship of the utterances of the one to the other arises. ... But a conversation also allows breaks. ... The task is to get to know the genesis of such breaks. ... We must go back to the psychological and seek to explain what determines precisely the free, or rather involuntary manner of combination. In doing so we must base this on our own observation of ourself. ... The most natural thing here is to think of oneself in the state of meditation in such a way that a certain tendency towards the distraction of thoughts is present as an inhibition ... here it is a question of that free play of ideas in which our will is passive though mental being is still active. (Schleiermacher & Bowie, 1998, pp. 124–125)

Here we easily find intimations of the play space Winnicott—influenced by the English romantics, though he may never have read Schleiermacher—would, more than a century later, find so full of creative possibility for development and analysis: "The more freely we let ourselves go in this manner, the more the state is analogous to dreaming, and dreaming is that which is simply incomprehensible, precisely because it does not follow any law of content and therefore appears merely contingent" (p. 125).

This passage makes it clear that Schleiermacher had no simplistic walk-in-the-other's-moccasins, enter-the-other's-mind conception of empathy (*Einfühlung*).* Instead, like Schleiermacher's hermeneut, psychoanalysts note the ways we find ourselves bound and inhibited in our thinking and feeling with the patient. Thus we come to understand the patient's world, the language we speak together, and the sources of our misunderstandings. We engage in something like what he called "reconstructing the meditation," almost dreaming together, understanding how the other or we together arrived where we arrived. Schleiermacher's famous claim to know the author better than he knew himself then seems less arrogant and far more dialogic, fallibilistic, and capable of being useful to always-learning psychoanalysts. "In general," Schleiermacher noted,

> it is the case that the more someone has observed themselves and others in relation to the activity of thought, the more they also have the hermeneutic talent ... the more difficult the hermeneutic task is, the more its completion demands collective work; the more the necessary conditions are lacking, the more individual directions must unite to complete the task. (Schleiermacher & Bowie, 1998, p. 128)

---

* This is also clear even in the passage often used to support the more simplistic view: "The divinatory method is the one in which one, *so to speak*, transforms oneself into the other person and tries to understand the individual element directly ... [it] depends on the fact that every person, besides being an individual themselves, has a receptivity for all other people ... everyone carries a minimum of everyone else within themself" (Schleiermacher & Bowie, 1998, p. 92, emphasis added). John Donne: "No man is an island" (Meditation 17, 1839, pp. 574–575).

Similarly, just as a good exegete (biblical interpreter) needs other commentaries on a biblical text, we psychoanalysts benefit greatly by long experience and self-knowledge but never lose the need for consultation and collaboration with trusted colleagues. (We also see that Schleiermacher generally made an easy shift back and forth between understanding texts and understanding people; for him the problems and processes were quite similar.)

We have seen that Schleiermacher believed interpretation and understanding to be hard work and to require humility and fallibilistic acknowledgment of the limits of our understanding. From Schleiermacher we can learn, thirdly, a holistic attitude, that is, to embrace complexity and refuse the sirens of reductionism, constant temptations even for post-Freudians. The two current attractions consist in "evidence-based treatment" (the idea that all forms of therapy should be experimentally testable for efficacy) and the worship of neuroscience (a new journal is called *Neuropsychoanalysis*). The first attempts to justify the time and expense that meaning-oriented "talking cures" require as compared with psychopharmacology and short-term cognitive-behavioral treatments, effective as they may be for immediate symptom relief. The second appeals to psychoanalysts themselves who are easily persuaded that now, finally, our work is scientific because we know how emotions work in the brain. We can "see emotions" on these amazing pictures that the neuroscientists show us on PowerPoint presentations at our conferences. Cogent and elegant arguments against these reductionisms appear in a recent article by Irwin Hoffman (2009a). A Schleiermachian sensibility can also keep us focused on the psychoanalytic project of healing through understanding, if that is how we understand our work, as many of us do.

In Schleiermacher, for example, we find that an emphasis on complexity and context did not first appear with Wittgenstein and Heidegger.

> Every utterance is to be understood only via the whole life to which it belongs, i.e., because every utterance can only be recognized as a moment of the life of the language-user in the determinedness of all the moments of their life, and this only from the totality of their environments, via which their development and continued existence are determined, every language-user can only be understood via their nationality and their era. (Schleiermacher & Bowie, 1998, p. 9)

Here we find the clinical usefulness of the famous hermeneutic circle, in which every detail takes on sense only from the whole of a situated life, and we understand a life (or a text) little by little from its details. "Nothing which is to be explicated can be understood all at once, but … it is only each reading which makes us capable of better understanding by enriching that previous knowledge. Only in relation to that which is insignificant are we happy with what has been understood all at once" (Schleiermacher & Bowie, 1998, p. 24). Schleiermacher taught us to be attuned not to how fast we can understand, nor to a quick sort of mechanical matching between words and causes, but instead to the holism and complexity of meaning. He spoke of a "zigzag" between parts and whole. If I understand what he was saying, he would agree with the complexity theorists of today, who say that what is complex, unlike what is complicated, cannot be reduced to simple.

Meaning, for Schleiermacher, was like that. Again and again he said that understanding is not something mechanical, because no rules can be given for it, but more like an art. What it produces, however, is always incomplete, just as in our clinical work. "The successful practice of the art [of hermeneutics] depends on the talent for language and the talent for knowledge of individual people" (Schleiermacher & Bowie, 1998, p. 11). He could easily have been speaking of psychotherapy. We may have further requirements—in the realms of *phronesis* (practical wisdom), vocation, and ethics—but they do not belong to a fascination with brain science or technical efficiency. Understanding in context, Schleiermacher believed, involved understanding the unique individual: "The possession of the whole spirit of the utterance ... rests on the knowledge of the individuality of the utterer as their inner unity" (Schleiermacher & Bowie, 1998, p. 254). We cannot research, generalize, or subtract out this individuality, the "individuality of style" (p. 255) or "idiosyncrasy" (p. 256). Manfred Frank's (1999) work on style in philosophy has reminded me of the irreducibility of the personal idiom so valued in Schleiermacher's hermeneutics. A focus on personal style, developed over a lifetime in intersubjective contexts, remains indispensible to clinical understanding.

Again and again Schleiermacher reminded us that "from the point of view of the hermeneutic task it is not possible to consider the object in isolation" (Schleiermacher & Bowie, 1998, p. 144). His *Frühromantik* religious sense of the infinite could not allow him any form of reductionism and supports the efforts of psychoanalytic hermeneuts and complexity theorists (Coburn, 2002; Gotthold, 2009; Sander, 2002) today to resist temptations to rush to explanation, whether diagnostic, theoretical, neuroscientific, or otherwise.

Here is a brief clinical example, disguised and combined to protect privacy. One young patient had had no previous treatment but was the son of a social worker who had used diagnostic terminology and psychoanalytic jargon on her children. Having filled out the psychologist's questionnaire in the waiting room, he entered the consulting room for his first session. The therapist took the papers and began to read. Without once looking at the prospective patient, she murmured, "Oh, this is bad ... this is *really* bad." Before the end of the session, the psychologist offered this young man the option of working with her or of being referred to someone else. The patient, thinking at the time that "at least this is someone who seems to know something," stayed for a year. During this time, he was repeatedly treated as a case of one thing after another, despite his objections to the know-it-all (*Besserwisser*) interpretations and predictions of the therapist. By the time he left this treatment, his traumatized state of shock and confusion had worsened exponentially, and he felt seriously suicidal.*

In this state the patient came to me, and we have been working together for many years. It has been extremely important that our work include at every point the three elements I have been emphasizing in Schleiermacher: (a) the "strict practice" that assumes misunderstanding as the normal condition and works unstintingly to overcome it, (b) the willingness on the part of therapists and analysts to admit mistakes and to try to understand their origins in our own history and emotional convictions, and (c) the attempt we both make together to resist too much knowing and to understand everything as part of the larger picture of violence, invalidation, and domination in the patient's life experience—psychoanalyst Leonard Shengold (1989) would have called it "soul murder"—while telling and retelling the past and current stories that add up to this picture. All this occurs within the story of the ongoing and always changing connection between the two of us, which has included, as sometimes happens, a kind of emotional adoption. This patient has suffered extensive losses from complex trauma but has many gifts as well as a uniquely personal style that we have learned, Schleiermacher-wise, to understand and to treasure. He has become a good-enough parent and a more-than-decent human being.

HISTORY OF HERMENEUTICS: DILTHEY AND HEIDEGGER AS TRANSITIONAL FIGURES

Wilhelm Dilthey (1833–1911), the next major figure in the history of hermeneutics, taught Martin Buber (the rudiments of whose *Ich-Du* meeting already appear in Dilthey) and influenced the phenomenological hermeneutics of Heidegger and Gadamer. Best known for his insistence that the human sciences (*Geisteswissenschaften*) provide their own access to truth, equal in importance to that of the exact

---

* I also told this story in Orange (2009a).

sciences or *Naturwissenschaften*, he brought into philosophy the emphasis on "lived experience": "An expression of lived experience can contain more of the nexus of psychic life than any introspection can catch sight of. It draws from the depths not illuminated by consciousness. ... Such expressions are not to be judged as true or false but as truthful or untruthful" (Dilthey, Makkreel, & Rodi, 2002, p. 228). We can already see two important elements of his hermeneutics here: It locates understanding in the lived experiential situation instead of in some inner mind, and it refuses a dualistic conception of truth and falsity. It accepts ambiguity and assumes the intent to be truthful.

As a young man, Dilthey wrote the best biography that we have of Schleiermacher, then in his middle years he turned to larger and more general philosophical concerns, but in his last years he returned to the study of hermeneutics. In what is probably his most important work, *The Formation of the Historical World in the Human Sciences* (Dilthey et al., 2002) originally published in 1910, Dilthey claimed that hermeneutic understanding meant not reconstructing the individual mind of the author but rather, by way of the famous hermeneutical circle,* going back to the whole complex purposive system in which the text or historical experience emerged: "All these modes of cooperation manifest a life-concern connected to the human essence that links individuals with each other—a core, as it were, that cannot be grasped psychologically but is revealed in every such system of relations among human beings" (Dilthey et al., 2002, p. 176). For Dilthey, in other words, hermeneutics understands historically, that is, contextually.†

It is crucial for the history of hermeneutics that the young Martin Heidegger, in the early 1920s leading up to the 1928 writing of

---

* This is a key concept in hermeneutics, from Schleiermacher through Dilthey, Heidegger, and Gadamer. It means interpreting back and forth from part to whole and whole to part, because parts gain meaning from contextual wholes, and wholes can be seen, gestalt-wise, only from their parts.
† See Stolorow and Atwood (1984) on Dilthey in relation to the process of psychoanalytic understanding.

Being and Time (1962), was reading Dilthey. Having read Dilthey, he transformed Husserlian phenomenology and called his method in *Being and Time* "hermeneutic phenomenology," joining the two traditions.* For the early Heidegger, to be was to understand, to interpret one's given or "thrown" world as possibilities for being. We are "thrown projection," where "projection" means prereflective, preinterpretive understanding (*Verstehen*) of a situation in terms of one's possibilities for being in it. Interpretation is a further development of understanding in the direction of thematic, perhaps linguistic, explicitness. Interpretation thus presupposes a fore-understanding of the situation in which we find ourselves. Understanding and interpretation, fundamental modes or aspects of human being-in-the-world, had for Heidegger this structure of fore-understanding to be grasped through the non-vicious hermeneutic circle of whole and part. Meaningfulness arises from this understanding that transforms what we are doing, our everyday practical coping, by placing it in a new light.† But the truth itself appears suddenly, in a flash, like the earlier *Augenblick of the moment of authenticity* (Dostal, 1994). In the hands of Heidegger's student Hans-Georg Gadamer, phenomenology itself becomes hermeneutics, and understanding comes more slowly, though there may be "Aha" moments. All philosophy becomes, as it was for Socrates, understanding though conversation, *Gespräch*.

HISTORY OF HERMENEUTICS: GADAMER

Hans-Georg Gadamer (1900–2002), the subject of a chapter in my recent book (Orange, 2009c), returns here for a somewhat different purpose. There he appeared as an example of what thinking

---

* I am grateful to my collaborator and friend Robert D. Stolorow for pointing this out to me.
† Heidegger's view of meaningfulness, as well as his view of authentic being-toward-death, has been thematized first by him in *Being and Time* (1962), in the *Zollikon Seminars* with Medard Boss (Heidegger & Boss, 2001), and extensively in the work of Irvin Yalom (1980, 2008).

can do for clinicians. He provided philosophical hermeneutics to help to free us from our enslavement to a natural-science model of understanding in the human sciences and thus showed us an alternative to tempting reductionisms. Here we turn precisely to his hermeneutics—and especially to his emphasis on readiness to listen to and learn from the voice of the other—as a clinical philosophy.

It is difficult for me to write about Hans-Georg Gadamer without betraying the enormous affection I feel for him and my gratitude for what he has left to those of us who want to think dialogically and humanistically in psychoanalysis.* Thus, fortunately, in this context I need to engage his critics only en passant, because I have done so elsewhere (Frie & Orange, 2009). Nevertheless, I must seriously turn to his conception of philosophical hermeneutics and deepen the account provided in my previous book (Orange, 2009c). Only so can I show what is the main thesis of this book, *dialogic understanding, in a hermeneutic of trust, forms the hospitable response to the suffering stranger demanded by the ethics of infinite responsibility* that we find in the writings of Emmanuel Lévinas. Gadamer's hermeneutics made a radical turn—but he buried the change under mountains of Germanic scholarship, at least in *Truth and Method* (Gadamer, Weinsheimer, & Marshall, 2004)—from a concern with the contents and the methods of interpreting to the style and the spirit in which we engage the interpretive task. The style, seriously playful and dialogic, requires a humble and open spirit. So let us consider some crucial elements of Gadamerian hermeneutics that may be useful for everyday clinical practice. First and last is the priority of conversation.

Gadamer believed, probably mistakenly (Frank, 1977), that Schleiermacher's hermeneutic was too psychological, seeking to

---

* Already in 1979, Steele (1979) wrote extensively about the contribution that philosophical hermeneutics could make to psychoanalytic understanding, though he remained embedded in what Ricoeur (1970) would have called the hermeneutics of suspicion (see Chapter 2). Among those who make use of Gadamer's hermeneutics for contemporary psychoanalytic theorizing, foremost is Donnel B. Stern (1997, 2009).

enter the mind of the author. Likewise, he criticized Dilthey for what he called "historicism," for thinking it possible to understand a text or an earlier civilization through historical reconstruction, an analogous mistake to the one he attributed to Schleiermacher. Instead, he thought, we can understand only from engaging in dialogue with the other—the text, the person, the work of art—and expecting to learn from the other. The fundamental dialogic attitude consisted for him in this expectation that one had something to learn and should expect to be surprised: "Every experience worthy of the name thwarts an expectation" (Gadamer et al., 2004, p. 350).* Indeed, he claimed,

> We say that we "conduct" a conversation, but the more genuine a conversation is, the less its conduct lies within the will of either partner. Thus a genuine conversation is never the one that we wanted to conduct. Rather, it is generally more correct to say that we fall into conversation, or even that we become involved in it. The way one word follows another, with the conversation taking its own twists and reaching its own conclusion, may well be conducted in some way, but the partners conversing are far less the leaders of it than the led. No one knows in advance what will "come out" of a conversation. Understanding or its failure is like an event that happens to us. (p. 385)

So conversation takes first place in Gadamerian hermeneutics, and its route remains unpredictable, just as we find in clinical work.

The hermeneutic circle, a second element, remains important for Gadamer as for every hermeneut and appears frequently in his work. "Every experience [*Erlebnis*, in this context, almost adventure] is taken out of the continuity of life and at the same time related to the whole of one's life" (Gadamer et al., 2004, p. 60). Just

---

* Each republication, with revisions, of the English translation of Gadamer's magnum opus, *Wahrheit und Methode*, or *Truth and Method*, has new pagination, unfortunately confounding all who want to refer or find references and perhaps confirming Descartes's theory of the *malin genie* (the wicked god who deliberately confuses and misleads us). On the assumption, or in the hope, that most of my readers will be using the latest version, I will refer to the 2004 version.

as the biblical interpreters did from Luther on (p. 176), we read meanings part to whole, and whole to part.

Third, Gadamer's hermeneutics, while nonhistoricist, remains deeply indebted to both Dilthey's contextualism and to his insistence on the possibility of establishing truthfulness within the human sciences. We find him criticizing the notion of self-contained *Eigenbedeutsamkeit* (own- or self-signification) in aesthetics, a concept that suggests that a work of art has or "represents"* its own significance independent of context or interpretation. On the contrary, he thought, all "understanding must be conceived as a part of the event in which meaning occurs" (Gadamer et al., 2004, p. 157). The *Eigenbedeutsamkeit* resembles one-person psychology with its search for methodical truth and perfect certitudes, to be replaced by the back-and-forth dialogic process of understanding sought in conversation between worlds of experience always existing in traditions to which we belong. Meaning occurs. There is, Gadamer wrote, "something absurd about the whole idea of a unique, correct interpretation" (p. 118).

Fourth, Gadamer transformed Heidegger's existential *Verstehen* (understanding) into his own *Verständigung* (understanding as a dialogic process, coming-to-an-understanding).† Along the way, he revisited Schleiermacher's idea that misunderstanding is always more likely than not, at least a universal possibility. Gadamer believed that Schleiermacher attributed this possibility to the experience of the alienness of the other: "In a new and universal sense, alienation is inextricably given with the individuality of the Thou" (Gadamer et al., 2004, p. 180). Gadamer thought that Schleiermacher did not exactly see that this very alienation creates the possibility of dialogic understanding. When attempts to reach agreement are in vain, "only then does the effort of understanding become aware of the individuality of the Thou and take account

---

* For Gadamer, representation means "coming to presentation" as in an artistic performance, not a copy existing in someone's "mind."
† I grant to both Heidegger and Gadamer scholars that this oversimplifies the relationship.

of his *uniqueness*" (p. 181). In other words, "Schleiermacher's model of hermeneutics is the congenial understanding that can be achieved in the relation between I and Thou" (p. 233); only when it fails do we have the breakdown that Schleiermacher called misunderstanding and took to be our normal human condition. In Gadamer's own view, expressed once again at 100 years old,

> Hermeneutics is *die Kunst der Verständigung*—the art of reaching an understanding—of something or with someone ... this "coming to an understanding" of our practical situations and what we must do in them is not monological; rather, it has the character of a conversation. We are dealing with each other. Our human form of life has an "I and thou" character and an "I and we" character, and also a "we and we" character. In our practical affairs we depend on our ability to arrive at an understanding. And reaching an understanding happens in conversation, in a dialogue. (Gadamer, Dutt, & Palmer, 2001, p. 79)

Gadamer emphasized, fifth, and most controversially, tradition. He used two words, *Tradition* and *Überlieferung* (handing down), depending on whether he was stressing the content or process of tradition. Jürgen Habermas, Karl-Otto Apel, and others (Apel, 1971; Warnke, 1987) accused him, after the publication of *Truth and Method*, of having created a philosophy without a reference point to protect against falling into uncriticized political ideologies (again!). Gadamer responded that no one can participate in dialogue, including those necessary for civic and political life so valued in Habermas's emancipatory reflection, except from some standpoint that remains historically grounded. His emphasis on tradition reminds us to take our inevitable perspectives into account. "We should," he insisted, "learn to understand ourselves better and recognize that in all understanding, whether we are expressly aware of it or not, the efficacy of history is at work" (Gadamer et al., 2004, p. 300). For us clinicians, this means never presuming that we have a perspective-free view of our patient, or of what occurs between us, or even of our own participation in the clinical dialogue. The hermeneutic emphasis on tradition and prejudice (Wachterhauser, 2002) requires a deeper and more extensive honesty with ourselves and with the other:

> In reading a text, in wishing to understand it, what we always expect is that it will inform us of something. A consciousness formed by the authentic hermeneutical attitude will be receptive to the origins and entirely foreign features of that which comes to it from outside its own horizons. Yet this receptivity is not acquired with an objectivist "neutrality": It is neither possible, necessary, nor desirable that we put ourselves within brackets. The hermeneutical attitude supposes only that we self-consciously designate our opinions and prejudices and qualify them as such, and in so doing strip them of their extreme character. In keeping to this attitude we grant the text [the other] the opportunity to appear as an authentically different being and to manifest its own truth, over and against our own preconceived notions. (Gadamer, 1979, pp. 151–152)

Approaching the other prepared to learn from the other—the "hermeneutical attitude"—contravenes the danger of remaining trapped in the traditions to which we belong and the prejudices we inhabit. Instead, the interplay of questioning and being questioned opens the *Sache*—whatever is under discussion—"revealing the questionability of what is questioned" (Gadamer et al., 2004, p. 357). He often said that we can understand what the other says only by taking it as the answer to some question, a question that we need to find and comprehend. Indeed, in honest dialogue, we attempt to make the perspective of the other as strong as possible, respecting that of the other and risking our own (p. 361):*

> My own hermeneutical project is, with regard to its fundamental philosophical aim, not much more than the expression of the conviction that we arrive at the things themselves only in conversation. Only when we expose ourselves to a possible opposed view have we any chance of getting beyond the confines of our own assumptions. (Gadamer, 1987, p. 30)

---

* "Important is Gadamer's recognition that all genuine conversation, and certainly all genuine philosophical conversation, involves exposing ourselves and our conviction to what resists, questions, negates or opposes us and them" (Gonzalez, 2006, p. 330).

Granted, Gadamer's emphasis on tradition left him vulnerable to the attacks of those who saw him as unconsciously conservative and hermeneutics as therefore dangerous. Another reading, however, hears him according to all of us a history that we do not choose but that we must take into account if it is not to control us and to destroy our dialogic participation. Awareness of our belongingness in tradition resembles the insistence, in most psychoanalytic groups, on thinking developmentally. Furthermore, awareness of my personal and therapeutic traditions—as well as of my background of cultural, racial, gender, class, and other assumptions—keeps me alert to the limitations of my own perspectives and interpretations. Because my perspective is inevitably a tradition-formed perspective, it remains inescapably incomplete and always needs the dialogic corrective. To repeat, there is "something absurd about the whole idea of a unique, correct interpretation."

For us psychoanalysts, devoted as we are to the practice of interpretation, Gadamer provided a rethinking of the relation between understanding and interpretation. Though hermeneutic understanding was far more inclusive, interpretation itself, he thought, was always linguistic and verbal, contained within the understanding process, and made the understanding explicit. But he spoke intriguingly of the "disappearing" interpretation:

> The verbal explicitness that understanding achieves through interpretation does not create a second sense apart from that which is understood and interpreted. The interpretive concepts are not, as such, thematic in understanding. Rather it is their nature to disappear behind what they bring to speech in interpretation. (Gadamer et al., 2004, p. 399)

He seems at least to mean that interpretation does not add something to understanding or to practice, as Dilthey had thought, but just makes the understanding explicit. The concepts used to do this—in our work, examples might be transference, repression, or any other theoretical ideas—then just disappear in the interpretive process, as clinicians become fluent and experienced in their work.

> Paradoxically, an interpretation is right when it is capable of disappearing in this way. And yet at the same time it must be expressed as something that is supposed to disappear. The possibility of understanding is dependent on the possibility of this kind of mediating interpretation. (Gadamer et al., 2004, p. 399)

But perhaps he means more. I suspect that within the *Gespräch*, the conversation, suggested interpretations are proffered so subtly by both partners, most frequently in the form of questions, that they disappear into the ongoing process of emergent understanding. They come and go in the play, like the back and forth in a tennis point, forgotten in the ultimate outcome. As Ogden (2003) also noted, no one even knows who even originally came up with this or that interpretation—this is often my clinical experience too—and what does it matter?

Gadamer reminded us that *how* the interlocutors express their interpretations perhaps does matter, however. Too much force could overpower, overbalance, and keep the interpretation from disappearing. In an essay on the healing arts, he evoked the metaphor from Dilthey of the two-person tree saw:

> Our ancient text [I do not know to what text he refers here] on the art of healing offers us a beautiful example with the practice of tree-sawing. As one partner draws the blade the other follows in concert, so that the whole sawing process constitutes what Viktor von Weiszäcker calls a *Gestaltkreis*, an internally unified configuration in which the respective movements of the two tree-cutters fuse to become a single rhythmic flux of movement. And here we come on a significant remark which suggests something of the mysterious character of equilibrium: "Yet if they employ violent force, they will fail utterly." (Gadamer, 1996, p. 38)

I am told that pushing the saw *at all* stops the tree-sawing process. Likewise, if one of the partners in dialogue, the therapist, for example, speaks too forcefully, the interpretive words do not disappear into the process of understanding but may become forces of domination, triggers for retraumatization, blocks in the therapeutic process. Not that either partner should disappear but that the equilibrium, in an intrinsically unbalanced situation, always needs careful attention. Just as adults are giants to children, the words of therapists and analysts may carry more weight than we realize, and the equilibrium of the dialogic process will need restoration.

ELEMENTS OF A HERMENEUTIC SENSIBILITY IN EVERYDAY THERAPEUTICS

Since Freud named psychoanalysis "the talking cure," psychoanalytic treatment has been seen as language based. Recent emphasis on procedural and implicit relational knowing, together with phenomenological emphasis on embodiment, has vastly enriched this Freudian understanding, but it remains true that most psychotherapies are conducted primarily in words. Language, resonant and heavy with history, is its medium, and the participants inhabit it, as other artists inhabit their media. But analyst and patient cannot be assumed to inhabit identical languages or experiential worlds, and each must constantly work at reaching understanding by learning the language of the other. The primary language-learning responsibility lies, of course, on the analyst, but we often underestimate how much work empathic understanding requires of patients. We call the process of coming to an understanding of the patient's life in the context of the therapy relationship psychoanalysis or psychotherapy. Though surely not everything can or should be put into words, the attempt to contact the other verbally, and to express in words what comes to be understood together, forms the bulk, perhaps the core, of therapeutic work.

Traditional psychoanalytic practice described itself as providing interpretation of the patient's "material." Patients were to lie on the couch, providing free associations and recounting dreams to a mostly silent analyst who would occasionally insert interpretations that explained the unconscious content (according to the analyst's theory) of the patient's material. Now in the era of relational psychoanalysis and of infant research with its emphasis on mutual regulation, especially gaze regulation, the patient is more likely to be sitting face-to-face with the analyst or therapist, the setup is much less authoritarian, and the focus is on conversation and mutual influence. In contemporary hermeneutic philosophy, conversation is the primary means of reaching understanding.

Understanding, in turn, is receptivity and suffering. Contemporary psychoanalysis places heavy emphasis on the personal agency and active participation of both patient and analyst. Without minimizing the concerns that have led to this emphasis, I believe it requires balancing by an awareness of the receptivity and suffering inherent in the process of understanding. In Gadamer's words, "The principle of understanding is founded on an inversion; *what presents itself as the action and suffering of others is understood as one's own suffering experience*" (quoted in Davey, 2006, p. 265, n. 13, emphasis added).

Not only are we required to witness and to participate emotionally in the suffering of our patients, but, in addition, the process of understanding itself means that we place ourselves at risk and allow the other to make an impact on us, to teach us, to challenge our preconceptions and habitual ways of being, to change us for their sake, even to disappoint and reject us (Davey, 2006). Often this work requires clinicians to leave aside* their own sense of agency and competence for the sake of the other. Working in the dark and experiencing our vulnerability does make us miserable at times.

Suffering, in turn, seems to bring us face-to-face with radical finitude. Gadamer connected what he called "learning through suffering" with finitude:

> What a man has to learn through suffering is not this or that particular thing, but insight into the limitations of humanity ... the truly experienced person is one who has taken this to heart, who knows that he is master neither of time nor the future. The experienced man knows that all foresight is limited and all plans uncertain. (Gadamer et al., 2004, p. 351)

---

* Perhaps, as Lynne Jacobs (2010) suggested to me, this leaving aside is itself agentic, a choice, but for me it resembles Ghent's (1990) surrender and often feels more like Lévinasian passivity.

The existential idea of radical finitude has, for me, two important clinical applications for psychoanalytic practice. The first concerns what I have elsewhere called fallibilism, that is, a constant recognition of how limited our perspective on anything necessarily is. This recognition helps us to participate with our patients, in a nonauthoritarian spirit, in the search for emotional understanding. Second, radical finitude means that, though unique and important, we are small in the universe and in the enormously large systems we inhabit, and we are living in the presence of our death. This double recognition has, I believe, a double effect in clinical work. First, it allows us the freedom to play in the clinical situation, to explore possible meanings without feeling too committed to them, to make mistakes and recover with the patient, to learn from the patient, and to make space for the emergence of the patient's own sense of things. Second, it helps our patients and us not to take ourselves too seriously but rather to enjoy whatever gradually becomes possible, given the particular circumstances.

Recognition of our finitude can keep us humble hermeneuts. A great temptation for practitioners in the human sciences—especially dangerous, I will argue, in psychoanalytic work—is the desire to be an expert, one who really knows. An expert is a person who possesses a body of knowledge not readily accessible to the public and who is consulted, either on television or in private, for this expertise. One may have expert knowledge of a foreign political system, of a rare form of cancer, or of the intricacies of tax law. The psychoanalytically oriented clinician, on the contrary, is a practitioner whose expertise consists in Aristotelian *phronesis* (practical wisdom) regarding the emotional life of human beings. This wisdom is not a body of knowledge but a capacity for applied understanding of individual human beings in relational contexts. *Phronesis* is intrinsically particular—just as Aristotle would have said—to this patient, this analyst, this moment in this history. Relinquishing the desire for expertise so that we may acknowledge the experiential uncertainty of practice constitutes a huge personal challenge, I believe, for most analysts. To learn anything from experience, Gadamer believed, the hermeneut needed to be "radically undogmatic." We need to be full of humble, but not suspicious, questions.

A conversation that leads to a shared understanding of the patient's life leaves neither partner to the conversation unchanged. "Openness to the other ... involves recognizing that I myself must accept some things that are against me, even though no one else forces me to do so" (Gadamer et al., 2004, p. 355). From the beginning, the sense that another person tries persistently to understand, often placing the clinician's previous understandings at risk, surprises many patients deeply and gradually enables them to take similar risks. At every point, the shared search for understanding is transformative. The transformation sought by earlier forms of psychoanalysis (i.e., via interpretations delivered about the patient's unconscious motivations) was thought to occur because the analyst overcame the patient's resistances, while the patient accepted and worked through the analyst's interpretations. A hermeneutic approach, instead, sees interpretation emerging from the shared search for understanding. Unless jointly authored, it is really misinterpretation and misunderstanding. In other words, understandings are not conveyed from one mind into another but emerge from conversation and are thus felt as truthful.

In general, having sketched some relevant history of hermeneutics, we could say that a hermeneutic clinical sensibility includes (a) a strong sense of one's own situation—including one's theories, personal history, and personality organization—that constantly and inevitably shapes and limits both one's actual understanding and one's capacity to understand a particular patient; (b) a sense of experiential world or system: one's own, the patient's, and that formed with the patient; (c) a strong sense of complexity that resists all forms of reductionism and technical rationality in clinical work; (d) a sensitivity to the languages of personal experience, including their nonverbal contexts and forms of expression; (e) a strong developmental-historical sense that gives, overall, equal emphasis to past and future, that is, a sensibility that attends to processes of emergence, including emergence of defense and dissociation, throughout the clinical process; (f) a sense that understanding is application (i.e., that understanding in the rich sense is curative); and (g) a sense of vocation and devotion similar to Schleiermacher's "rigorous practice." For him, as we have seen, "misunderstanding occurs as a matter of course, and so understanding must be willed and sought at every point" (Schleiermacher & Kimmerle, 1977, p. 110).

THE HERMENEUTICS OF SUSPICION

Paul Ricoeur (1913–2005), the most important French philosopher of hermeneutics, contributed a famous distinction in his *Freud and Philosophy* (Ricoeur, 1970). Believing the field of hermeneutics "at war" with itself, divided primarily between psychoanalysis and the phenomenology of religion, he described what he called a hermeneutics of suspicion and a hermeneutics of faith or restoration of meaning. "Hermeneutics seems to me to be animated by this double motivation: willingness to suspect, willingness to listen; vow of rigor, vow of obedience" (p. 27). The "school of suspicion" included Marx, Nietzsche, and Freud, "the three great destroyers." By suspicion he meant not so much interpreting down or disparagingly, reading people's motives as if they were up to no good, but rather looking for motives behind a theory's claims to meaning: impulses, class interests, will to power. What Marx, Nietzsche, and Freud had in common was "the decision to look upon the whole of consciousness primarily as 'false' consciousness" (p. 33). Nevertheless, they were not skeptics, according to Ricoeur, but liberators. More precisely, these 19th-century* "masters of suspicion" set out to, in Ricoeur's words, "clear the horizon for a more authentic word, for a new reign of Truth, not only by

---

* Had he reached back further into history, I think Ricoeur might particularly have noted Niccolo Machiavelli, though perhaps without the same emancipatory intent, except from illusions of benevolence, even one's own.

means of a 'destructive' critique, but by the invention of an art of interpreting" (p. 33). "Beginning with them, understanding is hermeneutics: henceforward, to seek meaning is no longer to spell out the consciousness of meaning but to *decipher its expressions*" (p. 33). In the case of Freud, we see this method not only in his case studies but most explicitly in his *Negation* (1925), where he taught us to read every statement of a patient as meaning the opposite of what the person consciously intended to say. With Habermas, Ricoeur was the philosopher most responsible for making psychoanalysts conscious of our work and theory as hermeneutic.

But Ricoeur also made the *style* of the master of suspicion, including his clever psychoanalyst, clear: "The man of suspicion carries out in reverse the work of falsification of the man of guile" (p. 34). He continued, "Freud entered the problem of false consciousness via the double road of dreams and neurotic symptoms; his working hypothesis has the same limits as his angle of attack, which was … an economics of instincts" (p. 33). In other words, Freud's hermeneutics, his theory of meaning, assumes that consciousness always disguises and negates the truth. He therefore had to approach the patient via a tangled theory of underlying and hidden motives, what Ricoeur called a "mediate science of meaning" (p. 33). There could be no direct human-to-human contact. The school of suspicion assumes that the interpreter always faces primarily an effort not to reveal but to conceal. The hermeneut needs, therefore, what Ricoeur called a "double guile" in the attempt to outwit and unmask the motivated falsehoods and deception. What the interpreter seeks to uncover will be unconscious or at least latent. The hermeneut need assume not malicious intent but motivated concealment and disguised meanings. "*Guile will be met by double guile*" (p. 34).

Ricoeur believed that Freud, and the whole psychoanalytic enterprise as he understood it, clearly belonged to this hermeneutic tradition and that this hermeneutics of suspicion made sense insofar as all truth, as Heidegger and other phenomenologists had taught us, is both a revealing and a concealing, that things are and are not what they seem, that every perspective conceals others. He also, with Habermas (1971), believed that psychoanalysis intended to liberate people and, therefore, that the demystification practiced in its school of suspicion was undoubtedly necessary. To be helpful, the interpreter had to be a skeptic and to teach the patient to be a skeptic. Although Frank Lachmann (2008) critiqued such skepticism, he described it well: "One looks underneath or behind a person's actions to find the 'real' motivations. Behaviors that appear kind, generous, or perhaps even an expression of gratitude and appreciation actually conceal baser, unconscious motivations that are aggressive and narcissistic" (p. 4).

It seems to me that Ricoeur was clearly right about Freud. In his *Negation* (Freud, 1925), he wrote,

> The manner in which our patients bring forward their associations during the work of analysis gives us an opportunity for making some interesting observations. "Now you'll think I mean to say something insulting, but really I've no such intention." We realize that this is a repudiation, by projection, of an idea that has just come up. Or: "You ask who this person in the dream can be. It's not my mother." We emend this to: "So it is his mother." In our interpretation, we take the liberty of disregarding the negation and of picking out the subject-matter alone of the association. It is as though the patient had said: "It's true that my mother came into my mind as I thought of this person, but I don't feel inclined to let the association count." (p. 235)
>
> Thus the content of a repressed image or idea can make its way into consciousness, on condition that it is negated. Negation is a way of taking cognizance of what is repressed; indeed it is already a lifting of the repression, though not, of course, an acceptance of what is repressed. We can see how in this the intellectual function is separated from the affective process. (pp. 235–236)
>
> This view of negation fits in very well with the fact that in analysis we never discover a "no" in the unconscious and that recognition of the unconscious on the part of the ego is expressed in a negative formula. There is no stronger evidence that we have been successful in our effort to uncover the unconscious than when the

patient reacts to it with the words "I didn't think that," or "I didn't (ever) think of that." (p. 239)

Indeed, Freud's entire dream interpretation method (Freud, 1900) assumes that dreams conceal their true meaning. In general, the patient remains, as does the analyst, an interlocutor who cannot be trusted. Nor does this untrustworthiness yield to a straightforward method like "bracketing" the natural attitude, suggested by Husserl for phenomenologists.

Ruthellen Josselson (2004), who has studied the implications of Ricoeur's distinction for narrative research, quoted the player king in *Hamlet*:

> I do believe you think what now you speak;
> But what we do determine oft we break.
> Purpose is but the slave to memory,
> Of violent birth, but poor validity;
> Which now, like fruit unripe, sticks on the tree;
> But fall, unshaken, when they mellow be.
> Most necessary 'tis that we forget
> To pay ourselves what to ourselves is debt:
> What to ourselves in passion we propose,
> The passion ending, doth the purpose lose.

Conceding to Shakespeare, Freud, and Ricoeur that we are transparent neither to ourselves nor to each other and that we need always to be attentive to complexity of experience, let us consider for a moment some of the clinical costs of a full-on hermeneutics of suspicion. Above all, this suspicious, skeptical, and deconstructive attitude places us at a distance from our patient, and from our patient's experience, objectifying the patient and reducing the patient's experience to categories. Second, my clinical attitude may be teaching my patient to take this same attitude toward himself or herself. Third, if as a clinician I am too committed to the hermeneutics of suspicion, I will be distant from my own experience and skeptical toward it and thus less emotionally available to my patients and in turn more likely to approach them skeptically and with an attitude of veiled superiority.

The hermeneutics of suspicion also, as Josselson (2004) further noted, creates a kind of esotericism: "Nothing is assumed to be accidental ... only those who accept the fundamental premises of psychoanalytic interpretative strategies and understand this orientation to reading signs will find these interpretations coherent and intelligible" (p. 14). One must be initiated into the special language and be accepted as among those "in the know," among the experts. Even in the name of liberation, elites arise—think how difficult to read is the "theory" of many badly needed cultural and political critiques—speaking languages known only among the critics but meant to unmask the deceptions and pretensions of others. Traditional psychoanalysis has been like that, intending liberation but creating its own dogmatic systems and excommunications.*

As an interpretative system, the school of suspicion directs its attention to the gaps—indeed Freud used these as his most important argument for the existence of the unconscious (Freud, 1915/1953)—inconsistencies, omissions, and contradictions in the patient's story. The analyst may or may not be personally suspicious and may or may not intend to keep the patient on edge. But theoretically based assumptions that a question conceals a manipulation, that a gift hides a stratagem, that a "thank you" covers aggressive intentions, that expressions of attachment always hide sexual intentions do tend to keep patients at a distance from us. Even more contemporary assumptions based on more intersubjective and relational theories, where the patient becomes our opponent in a game of chess in which we always need to be anticipating the next moves, can encourage a strong hermeneutics of

---

* Once we enter the hermeneutics of trust, this "esotericism" assumes a different aspect: "It has been an irritating fact to its critics and an embarrassment to its defenders that the deeper aspects of the psychoanalytic experience may only be understood through intimate acquaintance with its practice. In other words, we can only know what psychoanalysis is in the same way that we know what it is to be human" (Reeder, 1998, p. 70).

suspicion. At the very least, we see the other as an opponent who aims to defeat us.

Freud thought his theory of the unconscious justified his version of the hermeneutics of suspicion. Though suspicion may not be cynicism and may remain a part of a devoted search for truth, its *pervasiveness* in psychoanalysis has, in my view, been harmful to both patients and analysts. Taken alone or even predominantly, the school of suspicion is fundamentally pessimistic. It would take more time than I have here to argue for this view, so it must stand as an assumption for now.

Before I turn to the hermeneutics of trust, however, let me say also that I believe the hermeneutics of suspicion, demystification, and unmasking to be both important and unavoidable. This approach teaches us to notice political speech that hides oppression and discrimination. It also remains unavoidable in any psychoanalysis or psychotherapy attuned to complexity and depth in psychological life, where we "suspect" that more is going on than meets the eye. I will therefore most frequently refer, as did Ricoeur, to the "school of suspicion" to signify its pervasive or predominant use. But I will be showing that for a humanistic therapeutics, suspicion must always remain nested within a hermeneutics of trust, where it becomes transformed into the questioning and risking of prejudices within a dialogic process.

THE HERMENEUTICS OF TRUST

Ricoeur originally* had somewhat less to say about the hermeneutics of restoration or faith (Grondin, 1994), except to contrast it with the school of suspicion, where he principally located Freud. This school of "rational faith," in the "very war of hermeneutics" (p. 56), belongs to the phenomenology of religion and seeks restoration of meaning. In Ricoeur's (1970) own words,

---
* See Chapter 2 for his later thinking influenced by Lévinas.

> The imprint of this faith is a care or concern for the object [the text or whatever one interprets] and a wish to describe and not to reduce it. ... Phenomenology is its instrument of hearing, of recollection, or restoration of meaning. "Believe in order to understand, understand in order to believe"—such is its maxim; and its maxim is the "hermeneutic circle" itself of believing and understanding. (p. 28)

Ricoeur did not suggest that we should abandon the hermeneutics of suspicion for this hermeneutics of faith and restoration but rather concluded his discussion of the two by remarking on our perplexity in the face of "harsh hermeneutic discipline" (p. 56).

My own endeavor, however, departs from Ricoeur's at this point while making continual use of it. Because I find an almost unmitigated and merciless hermeneutics of suspicion remaining, often unchallenged, both in psychoanalysis and in popular psychology, including tendencies to shame and blame the victim, I am suggesting that we attempt to describe—if not fully conceptualize—a hermeneutics of trust. My project probably would have proved unwelcome to Ricoeur, though I cannot be sure, because he seems not to have been acquainted much with contemporary trends in psychoanalysis. On the other hand, his friendship with Emmanuel Lévinas might have provided some interest in new forms of therapeutic response, as well as a source of the perplexity (always with Lévinas!) he himself acknowledged.

My own sense of a hermeneutics of trust finds its sources in my long reading of Hans-Georg Gadamer.* Gadamer scholar James Risser (1997) rightly reminds us that Ricoeur's version of hermeneutics differs from Gadamer's, which assumes a common world and seeks to find meaning within what Robert Dostal (1987) called "the world never lost." A profound sense of belonging—belonging

---

* A related idea appears in philosopher Donald Davidson's (1984) "principle of charity," according to which "if we want to understand others, we must count them right in most matters" (p. 197).

to world, belonging to conversation, belonging to tradition and history—pervades Gadamer's philosophical hermeneutics:

> There is always a world already interpreted, already organized into its basic relations, into which experience steps as something new, upsetting what has led to our expectations and undergoing reorganization itself in the upheaval. Misunderstanding and strangeness are not the first factors, so that avoiding misunderstanding can be regarded as the specific task of hermeneutics. Just the reverse is the case. Only the support of the familiar and common understanding makes possible the venture into the alien, and lifting up of something out of the alien, and thus the broadening and enrichment of our own experience of the world. (Gadamer, 1976, p. 13)

Schleiermacher's dictum that misunderstanding should be expected has to be understood within the hermeneutics of trust, the hermeneutics in which we accord to the other the chance to teach us. Because we live with others in a common world, we risk entrusting ourselves to conversation with others within it and risk reaching out to relieve their suffering.

Gadamer himself, 20 years after *Truth and Method* and 10 years after Ricoeur's *Freud and Philosophy*, wrote an essay titled "The Hermeneutics of Suspicion," in which he refused the choice between suspicion and faith that Ricoeur had posed, as Ricoeur himself later did, too. Instead he claimed that all hermeneutics, his dialogic hermeneutics of understanding above all, consists of and depends on participation in a common world:

> "Participation" is a strange word. Its dialectic [dialogic conversation in the Platonic sense] is not taking parts, but in a way taking the whole. Everybody who participates in something does not take something away, so that the others cannot have it. The opposite is true: by sharing, by our participating in the things in which we are participating, we enrich them; they do not become smaller, but larger. The whole life of tradition consists exactly in this enrichment so that life is our culture and our past: the whole inner store of our lives is always extending by participating. (Gadamer, 1984, p. 64)

This participatory sense of inclusion and welcome creates a sense that one's questions and thoughts will be treated with respect and hospitality. A climate and style of trust permeates this hermeneutics. British philosopher and Schleiermacher translator Andrew Bowie (2002) noted that Gadamer's whole approach can "serve as a reminder that in many situations the detail of philosophical disagreement is less important than *the preparedness to see that the other may well have a point one has failed to grasp*, and the disagreement may be less important than what is shared by the interlocutors" (p. 2, emphasis added). This attitude, so characteristic of Gadamer, places him as the central philosophical voice of a hermeneutics of trust.

This hermeneutics, further, intends to understand on the assumption that the person—as Shakespeare's player king says—believes in the truth of what he or she is saying. Scrutiny occurs within an atmosphere of trust. In Josselson's (2004) words, "We assume that the participant is the expert on his or her own experience and is able and willing to share meanings" (p. 5). To paraphrase Gadamer in his famous 1981 encounter with Derrida (Michelfelder & Palmer, 1989), we count on the goodwill of both participants in the dialogue as we search for meaning and truth. Furthermore, we expect meaning to be both transparent and hidden, both there to be discovered and emergent from the dialogic process.

We need look no further than Freud's (1952) case of Dora to see the contrast between the hermeneutics of suspicion and the hermeneutics of trust. First, let us note that Dora sought earnestly to get everyone concerned to take her seriously. Still, Freud assumed throughout his account, and presumably throughout the treatment, that everything Dora said meant something else besides what she said it did. (For a splendid example of how things might have turned out otherwise with a different hermeneutic, see Paul Ornstein's, 2005 imagined reanalysis of Dora.)

The hermeneutics of trust does not presume, of course, that the patient will be able to trust us as therapists or analysts, given the background of betrayal and violence that often brings our patients into our care. Instead this hermeneutics concerns a set of attitudes and values toward our work and toward the suffering strangers who come to us. These attitudes can create a climate in which they may learn—often for the first time—that some parts of the human world are safe to trust and that they can trust their own experience of that world. It is up to the everyday practitioner of this hermeneutics of trust to treat the lost and alienated stranger as one who already belongs to our common world.

At the very least, as Gadamer often said, we listen to the other, expecting that we might learn something and be changed by the other. This critical faith also shares with the hermeneutics of Gadamer an orientation to truth as disclosure, so that being questioned by each other in dialogue becomes our access to what both Augustine and Gadamer called the *verbum interius*, the inner word "that is never spoken but nevertheless resounds in everything that is said" (Grondin, 1994, p. 119; cf. Gadamer et al., 2004, pp. 421–422).* This kind of hermeneutics rests on the assumption that we share with the other, for better and for worse, a common inherited world (Dostal, 1987) within which we attempt to understand whatever we attempt to understand. This is the hermeneutics of trust that I will be illustrating in the courageous psychoanalysts who show up later in this book. It is a kind of *faithfulness* to the other and to the therapeutic task that links with the ethics of Lévinas that I will introduce in the next chapter.

---

* Gadamer (1973/1993): "What is stated is not everything. The unsaid is what first makes what is stated into a word that can reach us" (p. 504).

2

The Suffering Stranger and the Hermeneutics of Trust

One must lose oneself in order to find oneself.

—**Gadamer**

Who am I, so inconstant, that notwithstanding *you count on me?*

—**Ricoeur**

Trust transforms the pregiven into a ground.

—**Bubner**

Our journey through the history of hermeneutics has brought us to a crossroads. At this point we will pick up what some might call an ethical path for clinical work. It appears first in the hermeneutics of trust only vaguely suggested by Ricoeur, as we have seen, but later more clearly explained in his encounter with Lévinas. Second, we discern this trail in the gentle and generous, though always questioning, dialogic hermeneutics of Gadamer, in his attentiveness to the specific and characteristic voice of the other. Finally, in a very different tonality, and above all, the Lévinasian "face" commands me to respond, or at least not to kill; the face holds me hostage. These three come together, if not seamlessly then at least adequately, to form a clinical philosophy quite alternative to that originally taught to most of us in our training but well illustrated by the five extraordinary clinician hermeneuts we will study later in this book.

THE HERMENEUTICS OF TRUST

Here we need only to resummarize the idea of the hermeneutics of trust. This approach to clinical practice interprets from a point of view that assumes a common world, in which both people live, suffer, play, and search for meaning together. It assumes the goodwill of both partners in the search for meaning and truth. It assumes not that everything is obvious, explicit, and transparent but that what is unhidden also contains important truth. The hermeneutics of trust works from what both partners hold in common to find understanding where differences exist. It assumes, in a word, truthfulness and good intentions, in both or all partners to a conversation or interpretive process. Without this assumption, there can be no real dialogue.

As a clinical philosophy, this hermeneutic keeps us closer to our patient's perspective and permits an emotional availability (Orange, 1995) that heavy reliance on the hermeneutics of suspicion (see Chapter 1) precludes.* It gives us some chance to mitigate both the shame built into the psychotherapeutic situation (Orange, 2008b) and that particular to this patient, for we too may seem to have human frailties and vulnerabilities that we too are placing at risk (Jaenicke, 2008). The hermeneutics of trust invites less defensiveness, as it understands resistance and defense as absolutely needed modes of coping with unbearable traumatic terrors and lonely anxieties. Gradually such a hermeneutics makes a relational home (Stolorow, 2007) for previously unwitnessed traumatic experience.

Critics of a more compassionate psychoanalysis have always feared the loss of the detailed questioning so beloved in

---

* When I use Ricoeur's expression "school of suspicion," I will be referring to a preponderant reliance on the methods of unmasking of defenses and disguises.

interpersonal psychoanalysis and with it a needed critique and challenge to the patient. Mitchell (1986), for example, expressing concern about Kohutian and Winnicottian views, cautioned that "a receptive, unquestioning approach misses the function of the narcissistic integrations in perpetuating old object ties, and runs the risk of consolidating them" (p. 125). Note that Mitchell assumed that "receptive" and "unquestioning" attitudes go together. It seems to me, instead, that a receptive attitude, one that establishes the secure holding environment that a hermeneutics of trust creates, makes room gradually for all the questions that Mitchell would have wanted to ask.

Within the hermeneutics of trust, then, the questions beloved in the school of suspicion can find their secondary place. Once the patient realizes that the therapist or analyst refuses the investigator/prosecutor role, new questions often emerge: What am I doing to make this happen over and over again? A shared world of meaning and trust more or less established, it no longer matters much who raises these inquiries, and they often come from the patient. Depending on the particular situation, the clinician may also be able to ask, Do you have some mixed feelings about this person? But if these inquiries are too disturbing to trust, we leave them for the moment and attend first to the "one thing necessary," the state of the connection between us. The hermeneutics of trust does not mean that we can take the patient's trust in us for granted; as clinicians, we understand that trust is a fragile treasure—if not a completely impossible thought—for most of our patients, sometimes found only after many years of treatment.*

---

* From Hans-Georg Gadamer (1996): "On the other hand [versus scientific medical techniques], there remains what we call treatment. The German term *Behandlung* is a rich and significant word for 'treating' people and 'handling' them with care. Within it one hears literally the word 'hand,' the skilled and practiced hand that can recognize problems simply through feeling and touching the affected parts of the patient's body. 'Treatment' in this sense is something which goes far beyond mere progress in modern techniques. Here it is not only a question of the skilled hand but of the sensitive ear which is attentive to the significance of what the patient says, and of the doctor's observant and unobtrusive eye which knows how to protect the patient from unnecessary distress" (p. 99).

40 • The Suffering Stranger

The hermeneutics of trust principally concerns our attitude toward our patients: trusting that they are trying to communicate their truth to us, by whatever they are saying or doing, and that it is up to us to try to understand. Until the patient actually attacks me physically, or until the relentless contempt becomes more than I can bear (Orange, 2009b), I give my patient the benefit of the doubt, on the assumption that he or she is trying to tell me something.

Although Ricoeur would have none of Gadamer's conversational hermeneutics (Gonzalez, 2006), we will see that a hermeneutics of trust weaves easily into Gadamer's dialogic hermeneutics and even more easily into Lévinasian ethics.

THE VOICE OF THE OTHER

Gadamer's hermeneutics, though extensively developed in relation to the literary and visual arts, contains a running auditory reference to the voice. He had a special love for Augustine's "inner word" or *verbum interius* (Grondin, 1994; Grondin & Weinsheimer, 2003). Gadamer's lifelong immersion in Platonic studies prepared him to understand this internal voice not as a solitary univocal subjectivity but as dialogically constituted. This hermeneutics of the voice, therefore, shows up preeminently in Gadamer, throughout his work, as a hermeneutics of the voice of the other (Risser, 1997). This emphasis distinguishes his work clearly from that of Heidegger, in whom the other disappears into Being, and brings him closer to Ricoeur, for whom his more trusting hermeneutic concerns the restoration of the meaning of what we seek to understand. Gadamer (1979b), in fact, actually described hermeneutics,

> To let what seems to be far and alienated speak again. But in all the effort to bring the far near … we should never forget that the ultimate justification or end is to bring it near so that it speaks in a new voice. Moreover, it should speak not only in a new voice but in a clearer voice. (p. 83)

Immediately we notice that hearing the voice of the other does not mean assimilating or appropriating it to my own. Dialogue, in Gadamer's sense, makes clearer just what belongs to the other's voice. His fusion of horizons (*Horizontsverschmelzung*) does not threaten the uniqueness and individuality of the other; instead, it seeks to clarify the other's voice in the process of inclusion.

Gadamerian hermeneutics invites the other to conversation (*Gespräch*), perhaps his favorite word and favorite activity in the end of his very long life. His version of Socratic "recollection"—for Plato, knowing meant remembering—was "not only that of the individual soul but always that of the 'spirit who would like to unite us'—we who are a conversation" (Michelfelder & Palmer, 1989, p. 110).

Whether we encounter a text or a person—in Gadamer's hermeneutics, the process of understanding is dialogic in either case—we meet the other precisely as other:

> A person trying to understand something will not resign himself from the start to relying on his own accidental fore-meanings, ignoring as consistently and stubbornly as possible the actual meaning of the text until the latter becomes so persistently audible that it breaks through what the interpreter imagines it to be. Rather, a person trying to understand a text is rather prepared for it to tell him something. That is why a hermeneutically trained consciousness must be sensitive to the other of the text from the beginning. (Gadamer, Weinsheimer, & Marshall, 2004, p. 271)

This passage could serve as an introduction to clinical practice. Every hour of our day we try to resist fitting our patient into our preconceived ideas and to listen to the person who struggles to give voice to his or her confusion, suffering, hopes, and despair. Unfortunately Gadamer himself agreed with Ricoeur that psychoanalytic work exemplified the hermeneutics of suspicion (Gadamer, 1982; Gadamer et al., 2004). In Risser's (1997) words, "The therapeutic model is assumed to be hierarchical and non-dialogical as in psychoanalysis where the therapist/analyst is not a true partner in conversation. There are of course other therapeutic models"

(p. 252, n. 48). Fortunately we can say to both Gadamer and Risser that—thanks in part to the courageous people discussed later in this book—forms of psychoanalysis, as well as other humanistic psychotherapies, have now emerged that are truly dialogical and asymmetrical only in inescapable ways that relate to ethical responsibility. Many of us now share with Gadamer a passion to make the voice of the other audible and as clear as possible, so that we can render it back to the speaker as his or her own.

But Gadamer knew well that the project of hearing the other's voice would often mean hearing what we might not want to hear. He wrote that we must be ready to hear the claim of the other against us, against the one who seeks to understand:

> Every encounter with others ... means the "suspension" of one's own prejudices, whether this involves another person through whom one learns one's own nature and limits, or an encounter with a work of art ... or a text: always something more is demanded than to "understand the other," that is to seek and acknowledge the immanent coherence contained within the meaning-claim of the other. A further invitation is always implied. Like an infinite idea, what is also implied is a transcendental demand for coherence in which the ideal of truth is located. But this requires a readiness to recognize the other as potentially right and to let him or it prevail against me. (1979a, p. 108)

What my patient is suffering, for example, may challenge cherished beliefs and emotional convictions (Orange, 1995) that organize my experience and keep me intact. My antidogmatism, hard-won and very precious to me, may be challenged by the pain of a young patient torn apart between a fundamentalist family and her studies in philosophy or science. I will be tempted quickly to dismiss the dogmatic religion and thus refuse to suffer and understand and undergo the situation with my patient.

In addition, patients' sources of suffering may evoke our own and threaten to retraumatize us. If there was bigotry, or sarcasm, or cruelty in our own families, it may be very difficult for us to work with patients we find bigoted, sarcastic, or cruel toward us.

Unless, however, I can receive and engage with such a patient, there is no chance for a healing understanding to emerge. Feeling that I already "know" this person, I cannot hear the underlying distress or its sources. An involved hermeneutic requires me to give up this knowing.

We can also think of this politically, as we hear the voices of people whom Europeans and North Americans have exploited. We may hear the silenced voices of the trauma of slavery in our African American sisters and brothers (Gump, 2010), for example. We will often hear it clinically, if, with Ferenczi, Kohut, and Brandchaft (see later chapters), we listen to our patients accuse us of misunderstanding and hypocrisy. We will need at the very least, in a dialogical spirit, to suspend our attachment to our desire to be right, our assumptions about patients' pathologies, our presuppositions about ourselves, many concepts taught to us in our training, or even the latest popular jargon in the journals of our professional communities if we are to hear the voice of the other, to "recognize the other as potentially right," and to let him or her prevail against us.

Working dialogically risks, as Winnicott quoted from T. S. Eliot, "not less than everything" (Rodman, 2003).

THE GROUND OF TRUST IN HERMENEUTIC DIALOGUE

What, we may ask, makes it reasonable to relegate the hermeneutics of suspicion to a secondary place and to trust the emergence of emotional truthfulness in therapeutic dialogue (including the nonverbal)? Gadamer relied on Dilthey's concept of *Wirkung* (effect), incorporated into his own idea of *Wirkungsgeschichte* (history of effects) to explain that we depend on our involvement in ongoing tradition. By this he meant not just thinking and doing what has always been thought and done but something more like what today we call "transgenerational transmission" of experience. As phenomenologist Rüdiger Bubner (1994) put it, for a hermeneut—and clearly here we see that every clinician functions hermeneutically, consciously or not—"it is important to school the ear for this phenomenon" (p. 77). In contrast to those who see tradition as imprisoning us, Bubner, like psychoanalytic developmentalists, saw it as giving us ground for understanding and expanding horizons:

> Being involved in tradition does not mean just being bound to the particular determination of a situation, but also means being confronted by an inexhaustible richness of possibilities. The hermeneutical activity of expanding horizons and stepping beyond limits, which makes up our true existence, unfolds itself by proceeding from a particular point of concrete involvement in tradition. *We are ourselves when we find ourselves at work trying to determine our reality* in argument with the cosmos of hermeneutical understanding. The possibility to do this, however, is given through tradition that engages us. (p. 78, emphasis added)

Gadamerian hermeneutics does not depend on cleverness, or on deconstructive reversals, or on unmasking pretensions, but on an

> original trust in the realizability of the hermeneutical task ... nothing besides trust remains in the face of that emergence of effects, which in every historical moment has long since taken hold of us, before we could carefully consider whether we should have dealings with it or not. (Bubner, p. 79)

Let us pause to consider this stunning statement, written by a philosopher about the hermeneutics of Gadamer, by a man who evidently had nothing to do with psychoanalysis, about Gadamer who considered psychoanalysis insufficiently dialogical. Our only possibility, both men tell us, in the face of our thrownness* that includes what happened to us before we could carefully consider whether to have dealings with it, is to trust in a dialogic process of our emergent understanding of the effects of history. Bubner (1994) went on, *"Trust transforms the pregiven into a ground"* (p. 79, emphasis in original). He went on to speak of the risk-filled

---

* Heidegger's word for the unchosen aspects of our existence: our family, culture, genetics, social and economic class, and so on.

"advance on trust" that affirms our implications in traditions, "which relativizes our own being, knowing, and capability in light of that which it is not ... the ground of understanding, which is pregiven in history, proves itself to be a possession, which in truth belonged to us already" (p. 80).

This language of knowing, possession, and trust in a common world, however, gets seriously disrupted in the ethical philosophy of Emmanuel Lévinas.

LÉVINAS: THE FACE OF THE SUFFERING STRANGER

On first look, it might seem strange to find Emmanuel Lévinas[*] in a book on hermeneutics. But his rejection of Heideggerian understanding as reducing the other to "the Same" (to categories, to the known and objectified) did not mean that he rejected every kind of understanding and interpretation. As a Talmudist he saw interpretation, as he would have said, "otherwise," as blowing on the coals of the traditional text or as offering a drink to the thirsty "widow, orphan, and stranger." He too had learned to distrust psychoanalysis,[†] especially for relying on explanation and on theories of unconscious motivation. Still, his work offers a striking contrast to our ordinary clinical ideas of understanding and interpretation and challenges us to an ethics of response and responsibility to the face of the destitute other. This "face"—not something one can touch but something that speaks: "You shall not commit murder" (Lévinas, 1969, p. 199)[‡]—unsettles any complacency or

---

[*] For an introduction to his life (1906–1995), work, and clinical relevance, see Orange (2009c).
[†] Hutchens (2007) would also dispute his relevance for psychoanalysis or for psychotherapy generally, but notably he lacks sympathy for the entire Lévinasian project and seems acquainted only with those forms of psychoanalysis that Ricoeur characterized as belonging to the "school of suspicion." To the contrary, however, important voices in American relational psychoanalysis (e.g., Harris, 2009; Rozmarin, 2007, 2010; Suchet, 2010) are now seriously engaging with the work of Lévinas.
[‡] It is "the face of the other who asks me not to let him die alone as if to do so were to become an accomplice in his death. Thus the face says to me: You shall not kill" (Cohen, 1986, p. 24).

knowing sufficiency by which we may be tempted. Thus, although respecting Lévinas's own sense of standing against psychoanalysis (Fryer, 2007), we can consider what his challenging philosophy might mean for clinical work that leans toward a hermeneutics of trust.

Lévinas, student of Heidegger and Lithuanian survivor of 5 years in Nazi labor camps, lived and worked in France until he died in 1995. He propounded one big philosophical idea, namely, that ethics is first philosophy* where *ethics* is understood as a radically asymmetrical "relation of infinite responsibility to the other person" (Critchley, 2002, p. 6). Lévinas became convinced that something "otherwise" than being or knowledge must be fundamental. In his first great work *Totality and Infinity*, he contrasted what he called "totalizing"—reducing others to objects to be studied, categorized, or comprehended—with responding to the face of the other.

This other, no alter ego that resembles me, bursts the bounds of the phenomenology Lévinas had learned from Edmund Husserl and from Heidegger. As David Ross Fryer (2007) put it, "Husserl discovered the other ego as an other ego like myself, but Lévinas discovered the other person as also a radical other beyond my capability and capacity to know" (p. 582). This irreducible "face" always transcends our concepts, representations, and ideas:† "The way in which other presents himself, exceeding *the idea of the other in me*, we here name face" (Lévinas, 1969, p. 50). The other (*Autrui*, the human other) presents me with an infinite demand for protection and care. The face says, You shall not kill (*tu ne tueras point*). You shall not allow me to die alone. Each face, in Ricoeur's (1992) paraphrase, is "a Sinai that prohibits murder. …

---

* The expression "first philosophy" comes from Aristotle, who used it to refer to his metaphysics, the study of those principles that underlie and transcend the contents of the particular sciences. Lévinas's point was that ethics is even more fundamental.
† Knowing and categorizing (in our field, diagnosing) reduce the other to "the same," to just another member of a class. For Lévinas, as his dedication to *Otherwise Than Being* made clear, classifying was tantamount to "the same hatred, the same anti-Semitism," whether Jews were involved or not.

Whereas Kant placed respect for the law above respect for persons, with Lévinas the face singularizes the commandment: It is in each case for the first time that the Other, a particular Other, says to me: Thou shalt not kill" (p. 336).

Lévinas (1981) contrasted his sense of the "height" or transcendence of the other with description or classification or civic agreements:

> The neighbor concerns me before all assumption, all commitment consented to or refused. I am bound to him, him who is, however, the first one on the scene, not signaled, unparalleled; I am bound to him before any liaison contracted. ... It is not because the neighbor would be recognized as belonging to the same genus as me that he concerns me. He is precisely *other*. The community with him begins in my obligation to him. The neighbor is a brother. (p. 87)*

Every reduction—by systematizing, classifying, pointing, even describing—is, for Lévinas, a violence, a violation, a form of murder. The neighbor, instead, exposes me "to the summons of this responsibility as though placed under a blazing sun that eradicates every residue of mystery, every ulterior motive, every loosening of the thread that would allow evasion" (Lévinas, 1996, p. 104). The response must be *"Me voici"* (me here): I am indeed my brother's keeper, and there is no escape.

In Lévinas's emphasis on belonging, though perhaps controversial among those who might accuse him of speciesism, we can hear resonances with Gadamer's emphases on belonging to a common world and on conversation, and also with the insistence we will find among our psychoanalytic hermeneuts that we are all more simply human than otherwise (Harry Stack Sullivan's maxim). Belonging in community creates obligation to the neighbor, to the brother, to the sister.

The relation to the other (*Autrui*) creates what Lévinas called a "curvature of intersubjective space" (Lévinas & Nemo, 1985,

---

* Lévinas used *autre, Autre, autrui,* and *Autrui* for *other*, without discernable pattern. I follow his translators when quoting and use other in my own text. I also include, when quoting, his own frequent use of italics.

p. 291). What can this mean? The ethical relation is not between equals but radically asymmetrical, that is, from "inside that relation, as it takes place, at this very moment, you place an obligation on me that makes you more than me, more than my equal" (Critchley, 2002, p. 14). Although we need law and justice and equal treatment ethics—as a kind of support system for the ethical relation—the fundamental ethical relation of proximity to the neighbor is so radically tilted and irreversible as not to seem equal in any phenomenologically describable way.

By "proximity," an important concept in his last major work, *Otherwise Than Being* (1981), Lévinas tried to explain what he called "incarnate subjectivity" (p. 86). Subjectivity, an "irreplaceable oneself ... is set up as it were in the accusative* form, from the first [moment] responsible and not being able to slip away" (p. 85). Proximity means that the other, right next to me, remains both other and separate but never allows me to evade responsibility. I am I only insofar as I am affected, accused by the need of the naked and vulnerable face of the suffering stranger. "In contact itself the touching and the touched separate, as though the touched moved off, was always already other, did not have anything in common with me. As though its singularity, thus non-anticipatable and consequently not representable, responded only to designation" (p. 86). Lévinas's language confounds, as he perhaps meant it to do, evoking the traumatic circumstances in which his philosophy took form.† He seems to have meant here that contact‡ with the other means meeting the radically valuable, someone beyond and above my attempts to predict and control and represent. In his less

---

* Lévinas plays with the "accusative": He contrasts it with nominative "I" subjectivity, all full of itself and also often repeated that the other's need accuses me, makes me responsible, even guilty in the Dostoyevkian sense that he frequently quoted: "Each of us is guilty before everyone for everyone, and I more than the others" (quoted from *The Brothers Karamazov* in Lévinas, 1981, p. 146).
† He wrote that his life was "dominated by the presentiment and the memory of the Nazi horror" (Lévinas, 1990, p. 291).
‡ He listed five words that go together, that also form major and minor themes of this book: "maternity, vulnerability, responsibility, proximity, contact" (Lévinas, 1981, p. 76).

strictly philosophical writings, Lévinas (1998b) would say that in the face of the other is the "trace" of the infinite, that "God comes to mind."

My response to the face is simply *"me voici"* (*hineni*), not "Here I am" as it is usually translated but rather, as Paul Ricoeur (1992) pointed out, "it's me here." The face of the other calls me, demands from me, takes me hostage, persecutes me. Response is my refusal to be unmoved, or indifferent, to the face of the other, to the other's "useless suffering" (Bernasconi & Wood, 1988). Sometimes Lévinas implied that I cannot be indifferent, that I am held hostage, but he knew very well that many do not and did not respond. This "cannot" must refer to the unavoidable ethical demand. What I am or need, or how I feel toward the other, is, for Lévinasian ethics, not in question.

Some aspects of Lévinasian ethics admittedly sound extreme, for example, substitution. Sometimes he seems to require that I be prepared to give my last ounce of bread so that the other may have a chance to survive or to volunteer to face the firing squad in your place. Working with severely traumatized patients, I sometimes notice that a background working attitude of empathic resonance or attunement, often playful in a Winnicottian sense, seems to break down. I find myself impelled to wish, and sometimes even to say that I wish, that I could take at least some of their torment onto myself, make it lessen at least for a while, to let them be less alone. What is this? Have I become a terminal masochist? Have I become a grandiose messianic figure in my own imagination? Should I quickly seek out another analysis? Or is there also something to understand here about the nature of our work, about the "therapeutic action of psychoanalysis"?

Let us listen to the formulation in his essay titled "Substitution" (Lévinas, Peperzak, Critchley, & Bernasconi, 1996): "It is through the condition of being a hostage that there can be pity, compassion, pardon, and proximity in the world—even the little there is, even the simple 'after you sir'" (p. 91). Robert Bernasconi explained that "this suggests that Lévinas is asking what underlies that behaviour which sometimes is called superogatory [commendable, but not required], gratuitous or as he prefers to say, ethical. His answer is that at the heart of subjectivity is not a [Sartrean] 'for itself,' but what he calls 'the one-for-the-other'" (Critchley & Bernasconi, 2002, p. 235). Responsibility for the other, said Lévinas, "is the essential structure of subjectivity" (Lévinas & Nemo, 1985, p. 95). In other words, according to Bernasconi, he was not preaching sacrifice but did want to account for its possibility. If we were as essentially for-ourselves as Sartre (2001) and others have believed, Lévinasian ethics would not be possible. Neither heroic behavior—like that of those who had risked their lives to save Lévinas's wife and daughter—nor everyday "*après vous, monsieur*" courtesy would be possible. We would live in the Hobbesian world of "all against all" or at least in the familiar "What's in it for me and my family?" world.

Rationality—the rationality of conventional morality—and Lévinasian ethics have nothing to do with each other. Clearly Lévinas did not appeal to the "reasonable man" argument of American jurisprudence; he never tried to reconcile rationality and ethics. Rationality knows, objectifies, calculates, represents, classifies, reduces, is always prepared to murder in the service of its calculated aims; ethics, as Lévinas used the term, responds to an absolute summons and command: Do not kill me.

Subjectivity almost disappears in Lévinas. Only in the suffering of the other, and in my response, do I (a *moi*, not an *ego*) come into being, "*me voici*," called into being by the other's naked and vulnerable face. The sovereign self, with its "place in the sun," always trying to have more, would be indifferent to the plight of the other. What minimal subjectivity remains to me, instead, comes about via my response to the widow, the orphan, and the stranger. Ricoeur (1992), in his encounter with Lévinas, spoke of the "modesty of self-constancy," so different from the "Stoic pride of rigid self consistency" (p. 168). He went on to ask, "Who am I,

so inconstant, that *notwithstanding* you count on me?" (p. 168).*
In the instance of a gift, "the other can be said to dispossess me on occasion so that giving is not an act, but an ethical event whereby I lose my sense of *mine* in the face of the other" (Critchley & Bernasconi, 2002, p. 240). Something happens to me in the face of the other's need so that my giving has the quality of participating. My background role becomes habitual.

More than 20 years after his Freud book, we can hear Ricoeur's (1992) much clearer preference for what we are calling the hermeneutics of trust, now framed in Lévinasian terms:

> Credence is also trust … a trust in the power to say, in the power to do, in the power to recognize oneself as a character in a narrative, in the power, finally, to respond to accusation in the form of accusative: "It's me here" (*me voici!*), to borrow an expression dear to Lévinas. (p. 22)

Now we can see how closely the older Ricoeur, the dialogic Gadamer, and the ethical Lévinas actually fit together as a hermeneutic for hearing and reading the more maternal,[†] and thus most often contemptuously excluded, voices in psychoanalysis. Without losing critique and questioning and concern for justice,[‡] we have a place for trust, welcome, and hospitable listening that places the need and the voice of the other first.

Freedom, agency, and authenticity have little place in the Lévinasian vocabulary, except to reject them (Lévinas, 1997).

---

[*] I am reminded of Bernanos, whose country priest without faith of his own speaks to the dying congregant: "'Be at peace,' I told her. And she had knelt to receive this peace. May she keep it for ever. It will be I that give it her. Oh, miracle—thus to be able to give what we ourselves do not possess, sweet miracle of our empty hands! Hope which was shriveling in my heart flowered again in hers" (Bernanos & Morris, 1937, p. 180).

[†] The complexity of issues and attitudes about gender—masculinity/feminity—and gender roles in parenting and clinical work—paternity/maternity—far outstrip my knowledge and the scope of my project. Nevertheless they have important bearing on the negative attitudes toward the clinical attitudes excluded from official psychoanalysis. See, for example, Vida (1997, 1999); Ellis and O'Connor (2010).

[‡] Ricouer (1992): "The sense of justice takes nothing away from solicitude; the sense of justice presupposes it, to the extent that it holds persons to be irreplaceable" (p. 202).

Apparently speaking to Jean-Paul Sartre (2001), who proclaimed that we are condemned to be free, he commented,

> The "for itself" as a mode of existence designates an attachment to oneself as radical as a naïve will to live. But if freedom situates me effrontedly before the non-me in myself and outside of myself, if it consists in negating or possessing the non-me, before the Other it retreats. The relation with the Other does not move (as does cognition) into enjoyment and possession, into freedom; the Other imposes himself as an exigency that dominates this freedom, and hence as more primordial than everything that takes place in me. The Other, whose exceptional presence is inscribed in the ethical impossibility of killing him in which I stand, marks the end of powers. If I can no longer have power over him it is because he overflows absolutely every *idea* I can have of him. (Lévinas, 1969, p. 87)

In other words, the face of the other demands of me a *subjection* (to Lévinas the only meaningful use of "subject" and "subjectivity") to the "dimension of *height* in which the Other is placed, is as it were the primary curvature of being from which the privilege of the Other results, the gradient of transcendence" (pp. 86–87). Sartrean freedom makes no more sense to Lévinas than does Heideggerian authenticity and resoluteness. "To welcome the Other is to put in question my freedom" (p. 85).

This surrender—not to be confused with masochism, as Ghent (1990) clearly understood—will clearly grate on a generation that grew up with European existentialism and with American therapies inspired by it. These words—*freedom, agency,* and *authenticity*—became our core vocabulary. These words also resonate with the emphasis on individual achievement, and independence from others and their needs, that American culture generally idealizes. Even for those of us inspired by the kinds of clinicians and ideas we study in the following chapters, it seems that we want to feel that we agentically *take* responsibility, not that we simply *are* responsible. Lévinas did not see those who do not respond as agentic, that is, as choosing not to respond; for him the subject is subject only as subjection. Instead, he spoke of *evasion*.

It is, of course, no surprise that renouncing our robust Sartrean freedom for solidarity with others will never leave us comfortable: "At least it will be recognized that this freedom [of the Sartrean for-itself, the I] has not time to assume this urgent weight and that, consequently, it appears collapsed and defeated under its suffering" (Lévinas et al., 1996, p. 95). At times, at least, bearing the suffering of others, witnessing and accompanying their trauma so that they may no longer be so completely abandoned, so that they may recognize the wrong that has been perpetrated against them, may give us the look of the overwhelmed. We are, according to Lévinas, exposed to wounding and outrage and infinitely responsible to the suffering stranger.

A gentler voice in Lévinas, more understandable and more bearable for many clinicians, calls us to hospitality in the intimacy of the home: "The interiority of the home is made of extraterritoriality [nonpossessiveness] in the midst of the elements of enjoyment with which life is nourished. This extraterritoriality has a positive side" (1969, p. 150). What Lévinas seems to be saying here is that to make a home welcoming, we have to be nonpossessive, nonterritorial. Against possessiveness, he often quoted Blaise Pascal, who wrote, "This is my place in the sun. The usurpation of the whole earth begins here" (Lévinas & Robbins, 2001, p. 53). Instead, hospitality

> is produced in the gentleness or the warmth of intimacy, which is not a subjective state of mind, but an event in the oecumenia [universality, generality] of being—a delightful "lapse" of the ontological order [of being, totalizing, objectifying] ... gentleness comes to the separated being from the Other. The Other precisely *reveals* himself in his alterity negating the I, but as the primordial phenomenon of gentleness. (Lévinas, 1969, p. 150, emphasis in original)

Lévinas accepted from Heidegger that we find ourselves dwelling in a nonpossessive, nonterritorial spirit in a home. Into this home, we gently welcome the separated other (the widow, the orphan, and the stranger) who reveals herself as other (this is alterity), negating me not as erasure—erasure means reducing the other to the categories of the same—but as "the primordial phenomenon of gentleness." In gentle, unobtrusive hospitality, the ego or I of the host largely disappears. Thus, he continued, "the idea of infinity, revealed in the face does not only *require* a separated being; the light of the face is necessary for separation. But in founding the intimacy of the home the idea of infinity provokes separation not by some force of opposition and dialectical evocation, but by the feminine grace of its radiance" (Lévinas, 1969, p. 151).*

In many places Lévinas said that *infinity* alluded to Descartes's use of it in his ontological argument for the existence of God— that which outstrips all our concepts. The title of his first major book, *Totality and Infinity* (1969), refers to the contrast of the infinite demand that the face of the other makes upon me with the murderous objectifications that he called "totalizing" and that he attributed to the entire Western philosophical tradition and to every attempt to know and categorize. Instead, the face requires of me both refraining from murder and the simple welcoming response of hospitality that he associated with the feminine.† The emphasis on separation points to his concern that the other not be appropriated or subjugated to the knower as the "same"; instead, the other remains truly a separate other to whom we respond.

ELEMENTS OF A LÉVINASIAN THERAPEUTICS: THE STRANGER AS NEIGHBOR

We should perhaps note that there are differences between what Lévinas, in his intentionally disruptive style, actually said and what we can infer from his thinking. A colleague from Australia

---

* It strikes me as a similar intuition that in Mendelssohn's oratorio, the Paulus, sopranos embody the divine voice. (The musicality in the Lévinas family, however, seems to have come from his wife, Raissa. Their son is a prominent French pianist and composer in the tradition of Olivier Messiaen.)
† Feminists have been widely and deeply divided in response to this aspect of Lévinasian thinking. See, for example, Chalier (2002), Chanter (2001), and Irigaray and Whitford (1991). It may, however, be relevant to the more maternal aspects of psychoanalysis.

wrote to me after a recent workshop in which many found the ethics of Emmanuel Lévinas disturbing:

> Psychotherapeutic hospitality has an essential psychological and emotional dimension. It is a welcoming openness of mind to the presence of the other's mind, in all its stranger-ness. We offer the hospitality of our mind: a willingness to welcome into our mind, and engage with, the full range of the other's psychological and emotional experiencing. It is with this hospitality of mind that we greet our patients at the start of each session, again and again ... over time, what is also importantly healing is the re-experiencing of this hospitality, and the sense of being psychologically welcomed-in—much more than tolerated, or selectively engaged with. It is a gateway to developing, perhaps, the capacity for self-hospitality. (Carol-Ann Allen, personal communication, July 10, 2010)

A Lévinasian therapeutics, thus, hospitably welcomes the patients and engages them simply, humbly, and patiently (Kunz, 1998). An understated style, attuned to the other's need and responsive to it when possible, will minimize the unavoidable shame our patients feel over needing our help at all or over needing specific forms of help. Recently, a training analysand, in treatment with me only for a few months, came to his session after a full day's work that had left him no chance to eat. After a few minutes of talk, he confessed that he was so distracted by hunger that he could not concentrate on what we were discussing and wondered if I had anything in my office that he could eat. He was quite aware that this was quite an unorthodox request to be making and that he risked not only refusal but extensive interpretive inquiry and humiliating disparagement. He also felt sure that I would henceforth view him as a "bad patient." Though he had not heard about Ricoeur's "school of suspicion," he knew very well the rules of classical psychoanalysis. But he was hungry, and knew me a little, and decided to take the chance. Once munching contentedly on the energy bar I quickly provided, he told me his many fears of asking, a long catalog of potential humiliations. The complex meanings of this request and response received extensive attention, though of course not possibly exhaustive. He told me later that he felt sure that without the easy provision of the food, we could not have explored the meanings.

Of course this simple story contains nothing heroic or esoteric, but it illustrates clearly the ordinary, everyday character of what Lévinas had in mind: that we respond to the other before we consider concepts, rules, categories, and so on. It is easy to imagine the discussion this example would evoke, even today, in many supervision groups, under the hermeneutics of suspicion.

This leads us to a second aspect of a Lévinasian therapeutics: its nonjudgmental character. It is not for me to judge whether the suffering widow, orphan, or stranger deserves my hospitality. Lévinas often spoke of the command coming from an "immemorial past" that precedes all ordinary time: "Since the Other looks at me, I am responsible for him, without even having *taken* on responsibilities in his regard; his responsibility *is incumbent on me*" (Lévinas & Nemo, 1985, p. 96). Incumbency means already in place, unchosen by me. There is no time for judging whether the other is worth my care. Furthermore, the other's need transcends me, is higher than me, so that I am never in a position to judge, for example, whether my patient *really* needed something to eat or not or should have packed lunch if he was going to have such a busy day. For Lévinas, that would be like saying that the other deserved to die for being Jewish, that someone deserved to be raped because she is a woman, or that one deserves violence or discrimination for being lesbian or gay. Just respond, and stop categorizing and judging from your high horse, he would say. It is simple to respond. *Hineni.* Take and eat. Take and drink.*

Nonviolence, third, would also characterize a Lévinasian therapeutics. Subtle forms of violence, especially those involved in

---

* Here we hear his reference to Christian liturgical words. Lévinas often commented on the resonances between the *hesed* (loving-kindness) of Judaism and the charity preached by Jesus (Lévinas & Robbins, 2001). While remembering that the perpetrators of Auschwitz "had done their catechism," he welcomed the papal letters around Vatican II saying that Christians had something to learn from their Jewish brothers and sisters, after all.

naming, would disappear from the practice of clinicians as they absorb this spirit. Technical and theoretical language, whether psychiatric, psychoanalytic, or from any tradition, tends to reduce by knowing too much and to keep the clinician above and away from the other's suffering. We will see that the clinicians/dissidents whose work we consider in later chapters, if they did not eschew jargon completely, sought experience-near language for their theorizing. Such experience-near language kept them closer to their suffering patients and reminded them that knowing was not so important as they had previously thought. It could even harm people.

Finally, in a Lévinasian therapeutics, asymmetry outranks mutuality. (Much as Lévinas admired Buber's work, he thought the emphasis on mutuality and equality missed the essential ethical situation; see Atterton, Calarco, and Friedman, 2004.) Friendship and mutuality, so greatly to be desired in ordinary life and love, suffice neither in extreme situations, nor in the doorway through which someone must go first, nor in the therapeutic relationship. In therapy—here Buber too recognized the indispensible asymmetry (Buber & Buber Agassi, 1999)—as in parenting, the asymmetry of originary (always already, "immemorial") responsibility often overwhelms the also indispensible reciprocity and mutuality, as Ferenczi was to learn (see Chapter 3). The needs of the suffering stranger are the *raison d'être* of the therapeutic relationship, and if we forget this, every kind of ethical failure can ensue (Celenza, 1998, 2010).

Three questions surface frequently when Lévinas comes into conversation among psychotherapists. First is the concern about the narcissistic and grandiose patient—so well described and understood by Heinz Kohut—who does not at all appear to be suffering and destitute in the Lévinasian sense. This objection generally comes from analysts and other therapists who value a more confrontational style and who do not really accept Kohut's understanding of the psychological fragility expressed in grandiosity and narcissistic rage. It seems to me that a Kohutian understanding and spirit will lead us clinicians to exactly the attitudes that Lévinas would advocate, a willingness to put ourselves on the back burner for a long time while we make ourselves available to respond to the suffering other. We will consider this kind of situation in more detail in Chapter 6.

A second objection comes from those who worry about the parentified child.* What about the patient, they ask, who has always taken care of others at the expense of her own self-development? Am I supposed to be telling such a patient to continue forever to put the other first? No, of course not, Lévinas would say. The ethical demand is addressed only to me. My readiness, my hospitality, my care for the patient (the widow, the orphan, and the stranger) changes the situation. This patient, little by little, remains no longer the person who has never been put first. What he or she does with this changed situation is not up to me. What is up to me is *my* attitude toward the naked face of the suffering neighbor.

In addition, this objection contains a subtle but understandable misunderstanding of Lévinas, who distinguished between my enslavement and my immemorial responsibility. In a very difficult passage, typical of his later work, he wrote,

> The psyche [the *moi*, not really I] is the form of a peculiar dephasing, a loosening up or unclamping of identity: the same [now the result of reductionism has been shattered] prevented from coinciding with itself, at odds, torn up from its rest, between sleep and insomnia, panting, shivering. It is not an abdication of the same [there is no organized I to abdicate], not alienated and slave to the other, but an abnegation of oneself fully responsible for the other. This identity is brought out by responsibility and is at the service of the other. In the form of responsibility, the psyche in the soul is other in me [no normal subjectivity this], a malady of identity, both accused and *self*, the same for the other, the same by the other. *Qui pro quo*, it is a substitution, extraordinary. (1981, pp. 68–69, bracketed comments added)

---

* Often a clinician, as many of us can attest.

Not enslaved to the other, the me, the psyche is at the service (reduced to "the same")* of the suffering other to whom it finds itself responsible.† The tiny homeless woman whom I meet in the passageway between the bus terminal and the subway every week on my way to work does not make me her slave, but she stands infinitely above me in her need for my protection and care, as do many others whom I do not allow to contact me in the same way. In relation to her, my imagined freedom disappears. Hostage but not slave: a small distinction, perhaps, but it makes the difference between a responsibility that one can carry as a hospitality, and one that rightly becomes—as Nietzsche well understood—resentment.

Third, there is the objection that when one loves someone, one does not feel obligated, taken hostage, traumatized, persecuted by the other, as Lévinas said. Surely this is true, but Lévinas was speaking not of intimate and personal relationships but rather of the widow, the orphan, and the stranger.‡ He was speaking of the patient I have not yet come to love, of the neighbor whom I watch taken away to the concentration camps, of the muttering homeless person on the subway. He was speaking of the man who threw himself onto the subway tracks to save the life of a stranger, of the doctors without borders, and of everyone who slows down enough to hold the door open for someone else. "*Apres vous, monsieur!*"

Finally, any patient whom I am tempted to reduce to "that racist" or "that hysteric" or anyone I may feel is unworthy of my

---

* Winnicott's (1949) hate in the countertransference, a similar idea, requires the caregiver to bear the objectification for a long time, until the patient is able to understand what the therapist or analyst has undergone and survived. I think he would have understood Lévinas's distinction between enslavement and resentment. Both advocate responsibility for the child, the patient, the suffering stranger.
† Among the aspects of Heidegger's early philosophy in *Being and Time* (1962) was *Befindlichkeit*, or how-one-finds-oneself-ness, which Lévinas valued and used to the end of his life.
‡ Philosopher Avashai Margalit (2002), on the contrary, views ethics as regarding duties of loyalty and care to the "near and dear," while morality concerns treatment of the stranger.

compassion or anyone to whom I allow myself to feel superior tests my Lévinasian convictions. How do I begin again—even when I feel besieged, persecuted, taken hostage—to see the suffering, the vulnerability,* and the destitution in the face of the other? For myself, I try to remember the "colleagues" we study in this book and to stay connected with my living kindred-spirit colleagues. (Other sources of physical, social, and spiritual self-care remain indispensable, of course.)

As I have begun to know humanistic therapists outside my psychoanalytic home—most especially gestalt therapists—I am thankful that many of us have learned to notice and to care for psychological fragility. In doing so, we have seen psychotherapy as an ethical pursuit. Far beyond psychoanalytic techniques and gestalt experiments, we are called to respond and not to abandon. The philosophy of Emmanuel Lévinas reminds us that this sense of vocation will always torment us.

THE HERMENEUTICS OF TRUST AND LÉVINASIAN HOSPITALITY

To ignore the differences between Gadamer's hermeneutic practice and Lévinas's ethics would be a mistake: (a) Both were Heidegger's students, and both worked out their philosophies in relationship to him, but Gadamer remained much closer; (b) Lévinas often sounded like a prophet on behalf of the vulnerable other, whereas Gadamer engaged the other in conversation; (c) Lévinas spoke the language of trauma and persecution, and Gadamer spoke that of play† and learning and emergent

---

* In the view of Michael Kigel, translator of Salomon Malka's (2006) Lévinas biography, "This reevaluation of vulnerability is the basic task of Lévinas's thinking ... a phenomenology grounded in an optical situation established in Auschwitz, established not by Lévinas but by Hitler" (p. xxiii).

† Alford (2007) noted that play is anathema to Lévinas; we might speculate that 5 years of dehumanizing captivity, together with massive family losses, could destroy the playfulness in anyone. Similarly Gill Straker (2007), who wrote from the context of the struggle against apartheid, speaks of "the trauma of morality."

truth; and (d) Lévinas thought suffering was the purest evil, whereas Gadamer considered it an unavoidable part of the human condition.

Let us nevertheless finally consider, without minimizing differences in their philosophical projects, the commonalities in spirit, attitudes, values, and emphasis between Gadamerian hermeneutics and Lévinasian ethics that make them useful to study together for reading the psychoanalysts who follow.

The Unique Other, Face and Voice, Is Irreducible for Both

Neither Gadamer nor Lévinas gives me any room at all to reduce the other to my categories. Gadamer's concept of prejudice means recognizing the inevitability of fore-conceptions in all understanding; his dialogic attitude means readiness at every moment to risk these to learn from the other. Lévinas reminds us at every moment that categorizing is downright dangerous: racism landed him in the Jewish section at Fallingbostel and countless others in Bergen-Belsen and Auschwitz. The voice of Gadamer's other says many things, so the interlocutors must listen and engage patiently, openly, and with endless goodwill. The Lévinasian face speaks too, essentially, only one thing: You shall not kill me. Both philosophers advocate, even require a hermeneutics of trust.

A Closely Related Commonality Concerns Their Brief Against Knowing

Gadamer's entire hermeneutic philosophy reads as a preference for open and dialogic learning over closed-down and possessive knowing: "The claim to understand the other person in advance functions to keep the other person's claim at a distance" (Gadamer et al., 2004, p. 354). Although Lévinas never spoke, to my knowledge, of hermeneutics, he often articulated a nonreductive signifying or "saying":

> The signification which animates the affective, the axiological, the active, the sensible, hunger, thirst, desire, admiration, is not due to the thematization one can find in them, nor to a variation or

a modality of thematization. The one-for-the-other which constitutes their signifyingness is not a knowing of being, nor some other access to essence. (1981, p. 69)

In his later work he often contrasted "saying" (the other speaks) with "the said" (essence, thematization, reduction to the same, knowledge, etc.).

Both Prioritize the Spoken Word Over the Written Text (Versus Ricoeur and Derrida) and Emphasize Response

Gadamer often said that he hated writing—he always felt that a critical Heidegger was looking over his shoulder—and he obviously enjoyed conversation to the end of his very long life. Apart from this personal predilection, he thought the spoken word had a living priority that the hermeneutic study of texts attempted to restore by conversation between the reader and the text. For Gadamer, a hermeneutic ethics (not a method or set of rules) commands me to listen with the attitude that the other may be right, that the other may teach me something, that some new understanding may emerge between us.

So both philosophers loved the written word, but both sensed the ineffable voice of the other in the spoken word. Had more humanistic versions of our "talking cure" been known to them, they might have disparaged our work less and understood our commonality of spirit with them.

Both Philosophers Find the Encounter With the Other Disruptive

Nicolas Davey titled his superb book on Gadamer's hermeneutics *Unquiet Understanding* (2006); I would probably have chosen "disquieting understanding" to emphasize the point a bit more. Gadamer and Kierkegaard both wrote of "the other who breaks into my ego-centeredness and gives me something to understand" (Gadamer & Hahn, 1997, p. 36). Openness to the Thou, Gadamer wrote, necessary for any real human bond, involves not slavishness but still a kind of surrender:

> Belonging together always also means being able to listen to one another. When two people understand each other, this does not mean that one person "understands" the other. Similarly, "to hear and obey someone" (*auf jemanden hören*) does not mean simply that we do blindly what the other desires. We call such a person slavish (*hörig*). Openness to the other, then, involves recognizing that I myself must accept some things that are against me even though no one else forces me to do so. (Gadamer et al., 2004, p. 355)

Lévinas (1981) likewise insisted that exposure to the other is not an active generosity but rather the passivity or vulnerability of "having been offered without any holding back" (p. 75). The vulnerability of the other makes me vulnerable, traumatizes me, takes me hostage, puts me in a state of suffering where the most I can do is offer my crust of bread, my hope from empty hands. The all-knowing psychoanalyst whom nothing surprises or really touches, held up to me as ideal by some of my earliest supervisors, merits inclusion by Lévinasian perspectives, among Shengold's (1989) perpetrators of soul murder. As much as disruption disorganizes and traumatizes early development—as all the psychoanalytic authors we will study have written—both Gadamer and Lévinas understood disruption of the comfortable complacency of our inevitable prejudices and places in the sun as completely necessary to seeing the face of the suffering other and to hearing his or her voice. We need to be upset to respond.

Disinterested in Individual Subjectivity, Both Are Willing to Surrender Self to See, Hear, and Respond to the Other

This follows directly on the previous point. Gadamer engaged in an extensive critique of the whole notion of individual subjectivity in *Truth and Method* that is beyond the scope of our discussion here and considered intersubjectivity just the pernicious Cartesian subjectivity doubled. For our purposes here, however, the ethical point is that if the other's voice has a claim at least equal to mine to be heard in the dialogue, to define what will count as important—as Gadamer would have it—consequences follow. Then we turn to Lévinas. If the naked and suffering face of the other stands at a height infinitely above me, all full of my comfortable categories and concepts and shoptalk, even more consequences follow. In both views, "self" is worse than a Cartesian mistake. In Gadamer, it frustrates conversation, hearing the voice of the other. For Gadamer, treating the other as an other means listening in a truly open way, holding oneself open, vulnerably, to the conversation.

In Lévinas, the nominative I, insists, dominates, objectifies, murders. The accusative "moi" is affected by the other's devastated face. (We must remember, as a biographical point, that although Gadamer survived the Nazi period by keeping his head down and avoiding controversy, Lévinas survived 5 years in the worst section of a work camp in Germany and lost his parents and siblings in Lithuania.) Both express an ethical responsibility; where Gadamer sounds haunted, Lévinas sounds traumatized.

Both Accord to the Other the Benefit of the Doubt

For me this informal expression articulates well the hermeneutics of trust. When the other's words and doings confuse and confound me, my hermeneutic of trust meets my responsibility to the neighbor's suffering in a way that Jurgen Reeder (1998; who notes his debt to Lévinas) tries to express:

> The Other is always beyond the reach of my knowledge, my fantasies, or my wish to objectify him. Faith in the Other is the sustained hope that I—despite his unrelenting unavailability—will meet him in his subjectivity. Faith shapes a prospective horizon that in its turn establishes a specific kind of analytical space, making it possible for the analyst to *await* the analysand. This kind of faith will in no way override or do away with the fundamental mystery of the Other—but it does offer a way of living without knowledge. (p. 74)

This "benefit of the doubt" attitude makes an enormous difference, as we shall see in the following chapters, to our attitudes regarding what has traditionally been called "resistance."

If we assume that the other suffers from situations that are originally not of her or his making but has developed patterns of surviving that now look somewhere between quirky and insane, we may be more inclined to listen more closely. We may hear the cry of an abandoned child inside the raging adult or to see the genuine despair in the face of the other who seems to be doing nothing for himself. The hermeneutics of trust emerges both from the dialogic spirit of Gadamer and from the ethics of Lévinas. Clinicians who need support for their inclination to give patients the benefit of the doubt can now tell themselves that they are relying on these two great philosophers and on a hermeneutics of trust.

Both Philosophers Embodied a Spirit of Hospitality, in Their Writing and Also in Their Lives

In Gadamer's version the dialogic person needs an attitude of receptivity to what is other and unfamiliar, an attitude that welcomes, he said, just that guest whom we were not expecting, who breaks into our complacency. Lévinas often characterized the response to the suffering other as hospitality. Gadamer, I am told, invited a former student to stay in his home during a period of his life that he might otherwise not have survived, hid and otherwise protected Jewish friends during the Nazi years, and was ever well-known for welcoming people into conversation. Lévinas quietly helped students in need, and his *Shabbat* table was always full of guests. This shared sensibility underlies the spirit that runs through the quiet alternative road we are about to travel. It leaves behind the strictures of "do not gratify" for Fromm-Reichmann's "How can I help you?", Lévinas's *hineni* (*me voici*, me here), and Gadamer's "welcome."

Both Unsettle Our Complacency

Perhaps this point is already clear, but it bears repeating. Nothing about the perspective shared by Gadamer, Lévinas, and the later Ricoeur leaves us comfortable. What an irony, that the hermeneutics of trust should be so much more challenging than the hermeneutics of suspicion! Nevertheless, entrusting ourselves to a vocation—called out by the face and voice of the other—means never fully being at rest. It means, as Lévinas often said, bearing infinite guilt* and never being finished with the ethical task. It means looking tired and persecuted sometimes. The other side, however, can be seen in certain photographs of both philosophers, where they are clearly responding to someone. Each looks luminous, as if he had seen something beautiful, perhaps the trace of the infinite. I believe both sides exist for us too, practitioners of the hermeneutics of trust.

PSYCHOTHERAPY AND THE RELIEF OF SUFFERING

It might seem obvious (Young-Eisendrath, 2001) that the primary and fundamental task of psychotherapy is to relieve suffering. As we begin our study of unorthodox psychoanalysts with Sándor Ferenczi in the next chapter, we will see immediately that no consensus has ever existed on this point. Freud himself took a greater interest in theory construction, behaviorists have espoused social conformity, and the existentialists have devoted themselves to personal agency. Because only the third of these seems to me remotely to resemble a human goal in the face of human misery, let us consider it for a moment before returning to our central project.

It is easy to see why a sense and experience of agency seems often to be equated with mental health. Infants, both research and informal observation suggest, take great delight in discovering that they can do things, can make things happen. Children and adults feel better, or at least believe they will feel better, if they can only *do* something about the problems and predicaments in which they find themselves. It might be argued that the most admired American

---

* This Lévinasian and Dostoyevskian guilt, infinitely demanding (Critchley, 2007) as it is, requires careful distinguishing from the useless "guiltiness" Stephen Mitchell (2000b) so well described.

attitude, apart from but probably related to, the lonesome-cowboy ideal of independence is a can-do, problem-solving approach. Even in international affairs, Americans often seem to value doing or "intervention" over conversation and collaboration.

But consider the alternative—the so-called victim mentality. Who would want that? Among several groups of the 9/11 survivors, for example, and among the families left behind, the popular wisdom was that the way to recover was to *do something*. You should get involved in airline safety issues, find out who failed and why it happened, support the "war on terrorism," and so on. Those who "nursed their wounds," or wandered around like lost souls, were not "getting on with it." They were blaming others for their troubles, not "taking the bull by the horns." Adults who find themselves still suffering from child maltreatment or neglect are often seen as "pathetic whiners." The contempt humiliates and retraumatizes.

Psychoanalysis, of course, until recently, went against this activist grain. The analyst's doing was severely restricted by the rules of technique, and the patient was cautioned against making major decisions in order to allow unconscious impulses and their derivatives to surface and become apparent. Neither participant was supposed to do much. Current relational thinking, of course, has changed this picture radically. The whole psychoanalytic process is understood as interaction, punctuated by "enactments" (Hirsch, 1998; Maroda, 1998a; McLaughlin & Johan, 1992), in which both patient and analyst are understood to be active participants. Now a sense of personal agency—together with its moral concomitant, a sense of responsibility—has become a psychoanalytic outcome greatly to be desired (Frie, 2008). We relational analysts and psychotherapists tend to value active participation—in life and in the psychoanalytic process.

I believe, however, that a hermeneutic clinical sensibility opens another perspective—one that neither is distant and disengaged nor makes us into action figures. The best name I have found so far is an attitude of receptivity, something I suspect is very close to Emmanuel Ghent's (1990) conception of "surrender." The longer I live with Ghent's idea, the less it connotes to me the pathological accommodation described by Bernard Brandchaft (see Chapter 7). Instead, I believe Ghent meant to de-idealize agency and to help us reconsider the kind of minimal subjectivity we find in Lévinas.

This receptivity, I believe, forms one of the most basic components of a hermeneutic sensibility. Neither fully active nor passive, it permits learning from the other and engagement with the other. In the beginning, this receptivity must characterize the analyst and can be very difficult. This receptivity goes counter to the mastery ethos of our Western culture, where the nurturing and the maternal often land in places of disparagement, to say the least. But our three strands, from Ricoeur's hermeneutic of trust or faith, from Gadamer's dialogic understanding, and above all from Lévinasian ethics, situate us exactly in this countercultural space. In Lévinas's (1981) voice,

> Where to be? How to be? It is a writhing in the tight dimensions of pain, the unsuspected dimensions of the higher side. It is being torn up from oneself, being less than nothing, a rejection into the negative, behind nothingness; it is maternity, gestation of the other in the same. [The other breaks into my supposed knowing that reduces her to the objectified same.] Is not the restlessness of someone persecuted [the accused *moi*] but a modification of maternity, the groaning of the wounded entrails by those it will bear or has borne? In maternity what signifies is a responsibility for others, to the point of substitution for others and suffering both from the effect of persecution and from the persecuting itself in which the persecutor sinks. (p. 75)

There may be many reasons that we do not really want to allow the patient to affect us so much. Suffering, as Lévinas told us, is ungraspable; we cannot dominate it. It breaks down meaning, at least until another responds.* Even more, he said, "The more I answer the more I am responsible; the more I approach the

---

* An eloquent voice for the attitudes we are considering in medicine generally is Eric Cassell (2004). See also Greenfield and Jensen (2010) for a more schematic approach.

neighbor with which I am encharged the further away I am. This debit which increases is infinity" (Lévinas, 1981, p. 93). This infinity for him had a double meaning: The suffering of the other faces me with an infinite demand but also places me in contact with the infinite, with the sacred, with the holy, whatever that may be.

But he also distinguished between useless and useful suffering, the kind he had previously described as maternal. Suffering itself, the purest evil, the meaningless condition of extreme passivity, constitutes the challenge of ethics, the task of medicine and psychotherapy. Its face accuses me:

> Is not the evil suffering—extreme passivity, helplessness, abandonment and solitude ... the half-opening that a moan, a cry, a groan or a sigh slips through—the original call for aid, for curative help, help from the other me whose alterity ... promises salvation? (Lévinas, 1998a, p. 92)

Suffering, however, displays that peculiar asymmetry that Lévinas called "a curvature of intersubjective space": It is meaningful in me but absurd for the other, unutterable. He thought theodicy, the attempt to frame defenses of theology in the face of unspeakable evils, obscene, and he wrote,

> There is a radical difference between *the suffering in the other*, where it is unforgivable to *me*, solicits me and calls me and suffering *in me*, my own experience of suffering, whose constitutional or congenital uselessness can take on a meaning, the only one of which suffering is capable, in becoming a suffering for the suffering (inexorable though it may be) of someone else. (p. 94)

For me this sentence contains not only the possibility of finding meaning in the bleakest moments of work with the most tortured souls who entrust themselves to my care, when I too feel nearly overwhelmed by their "useless suffering," but also perhaps a way to think about what actually helps people. Lévinas spoke in his essay on useless suffering not only of medicine and psychology but also of Auschwitz. Where others speak of witness (Orange, 1995; Poland, 2000), he spoke of taking on, of assuming the other's suffering, where it takes on meaning as a for-the-other. The overwhelmed and negated face of the other, he often said, says to me, Do not allow me to die alone. With protection and care, the other suffers somewhat less, and my suffering for her takes on meaning.

We could now make a comparative excursion into the religions of the world and consider their rich and diverse considerations of human suffering and ask whether they agree with Lévinas.* Though such a project would require a book of its own, few, I suspect, would dispute his claim that compassionate response to the suffering of others adds meaning to human life. What should surprise us, perhaps, is that such considerations have remained far from the center of the psychoanalytic literature and that the voices of those who have placed the care of the suffering patient before the protection of theory or status have been largely silenced. This book attempts to let their voices speak out.

A FEW NOTES

Commitment to relief of suffering as our fundamental therapeutic vocation has several corollaries, which scarcely need stating as they are so obvious, so I will be brief:

1. A compassionate attitude of suffering with the other is indispensable.
2. A dialogical, nonauthoritarian style is equally crucial. One can support without becoming an expert-authority.
3. Consistency and reliability, not a propensity to wear ourselves out, are essential to working with the profoundly traumatized.
4. We should expect to be affected by our work to the core of our being and sometimes to feel retraumatized.
5. We need our own supports, and sources of nourishment and hospitality, if we are to continue.

---

* Sandra Buechler (2010) recently compared attitudes toward clinical work, especially with respect to the analysis of defense, on the basis of attitudes toward human suffering.

Finally, it seems important to note that our ethical response coincides exactly with our clinical vocation to restore dignity to devastated, shame-filled, degraded, and suffering human beings like ourselves. In my view, treating the other as a worthy partner in dialogue—no matter what distress or symptoms the patient brings to the encounter, and no matter what aversive preconceptions the clinician carries or develops—creates the foundations for working within what we designate here as the hermeneutics of trust. Everything we can learn from every school of psychoanalysis and psychotherapy, as well as from other disciplines and from the arts, that helps us to meet and sustain the suffering other nonevasively, without too much suspicion, is both good healing therapeutic practice and good ethics.

3

Sándor Ferenczi

The Analyst of Last Resort and the Hermeneutics of Trauma

I started to listen to my patients when, in their attacks, they called me insensitive, cold, even hard and cruel, when they reproached me with being selfish, heartless, conceited, when they shouted at me: "Help! Quick! Don't let me perish helplessly!"

—**Ferenczi**

No analysis can succeed if we do not succeed in really loving the patient. Every patient has the right to be regarded and cared for as an ill-treated, unhappy child.

—**Ferenczi**

As discussed in earlier chapters, the French philosopher Paul Ricoeur has famously designated Sigmund Freud, Friedrich Nietzsche, and Karl Marx as practitioners of what he called "the hermeneutics of suspicion." They advocated and practiced "a method of interpretation which assumes that the literal or surface-level meaning of a text is an effort to conceal the political interests which are served by the text. The purpose of interpretation is to strip off the concealment, unmasking those interests" (Ricouer, 1970, p. 33). For psychoanalysis, this attitude particularly involved what Freud (1925) called negation, where the patient was taken to mean, unconsciously, the opposite of whatever he or she said.

It seems to have grown, gradually, from the point at which Freud "discovered" or concluded that his patients' reports of having been sexually or otherwise mistreated as children were only or primarily fantasy. An especially elaborate instance of this reasoning appears in "A Child Is Being Beaten" (1920), where he wrote repeatedly of his "uneasy suspicion" of taking what the patient said seriously, but there are many others. The interest served by the concealment or negation, described by Ricoeur as political, was for Freud actually defensive. The fantasy negated an instinctual wish that the adult patient would have found too difficult to bear knowing consciously before the analysis.

Sándor Ferenczi (1863–1933), Sigmund Freud's closest collaborator and confidant for 25 years, diverged from Freud's psychoanalysis in ways that still shape our profession today. Grandfather or grandmother (Hoffer, 1991; Vida, 1997) to most strains of relational psychoanalysis (Aron & Harris, 1993), to attachment theory (Bacciagaluppi, 1994), to humanistic psychotherapies, to developmental thinking in psychoanalysis (Young-Bruehl, 2002), to the primacy of clinical practice (or "technique") over scientific theory, Ferenczi is our closet ancestor, whom we only begin to be able to name.* His courage and integrity could not save him from his own intersubjective situation with Freud, as we shall see, but they may inspire us to protest in our own time against every form of dehumanization in our work and to reach, as he did, for any possible way to contact the suffering patient and to depart from the "school of suspicion" (see Chapters 1 and 2).

My immediate hermeneutic question, emergent especially from my reading of the Freud–Ferenczi correspondence (Brabant, Falzeder, & Giampieri-Deutsch, 1993; Falzeder & Brabant, 2000; Falzeder, Brabant, & Giampieri-Deutsch, 1996), concerns the conditions and attitudes that made it possible for Ferenczi to move

---

* Important books that seem heavily indebted to the Ferenczian legacy, but without attribution, include those by Bromberg (2006) and by Kohut (Kohut, Goldberg, & Stepansky, 1984). A major exception is Heinrich Racker (1968), who clearly acknowledged Ferenczi's influence.

from the language of "the hysteric," "the paranoid," and "the homosexual" to the intense concern for "the sufferer" and for the "suffering person" that we find in his clinical diary (Ferenczi & Dupont, 1988) and in the papers of his last years (Ferenczi, 1930, 1931, 1949a).* In other words, how did he shift from a focus on pathology to a concentration on the human being who suffers? I will be suggesting that he found his way ever more into a dialogic hermeneutics (see Chapter 1) of the relational situation and that it changed him profoundly. I believe, however, he was able to make this shift only because he was passionately concerned to relieve emotionally suffering people long before he met Freud and became so engaged with him in theory-building, and because he later met Georg Groddeck who himself embodied this passion. Thus in the end he was able to maintain his affection for Freud but could no longer maintain a sense of shared vocation with him.

Although I will refer to the Freud–Ferenczi correspondence (Brabant et al., 1993; Falzeder & Brabant, 2000; Falzeder et al., 1996) only as it illuminates the biography and the central later texts, it provides an indispensible context for them, and we can be only immensely grateful to those whose work and care finally brought this full correspondence to publication. Others have studied the story of the suppression of Ferenczi's late work (Rachman, 1997b; Roazen, 1975), and the various delays in publication, but that is not my purpose here. Still, these setbacks have also impeded our access to perhaps the most profoundly ethical[†] of the early psychoanalysts. This chapter, therefore, attempts to help us catch up on a shared developmental loss in our profession and to exemplify the thesis of this book that a dialogic therapeutics, informed

---

* Many have noted that this was his reputation: Aron (1992), Harris and Gold (2001), Maroda (1998b).

[†] I use *ethical* here not in the sense of bound-to-the-rules we commonly accept today—both Freud and Ferenczi violated these, most obviously in their discussion of the treatment of Elma Palos, daughter of Gizella, who became Ferenczi's wife. Instead, I mean *ethical* in the Lévinasian sense of responsibility to the face of the destitute other, the widow, the orphan, and the stranger, whose naked need places an infinite demand on me (Lévinas & Nemo, 1985; Orange, 2009c). See Chapter 2.

by the hermeneutics of trust, provides the ethical response to the suffering stranger.

LIFE AND WORK

Born to assimilated Hungarian Jewish parents in 1863, Sándor Ferenczi was the 8th of 12 children.* His family owned a bookstore, and his educational and cultural opportunities were deep and broad within the Austro-Hungarian Empire (Haynal, 1989b). His father died when he was 15. Sometimes described as his father's favorite, he called his mother cold and felt himself deprived of maternal nurturance. He studied medicine in Vienna, returning to practice in Budapest.

Ferenczi early took an interest in the marginalized of society. In the words of Michael Balint (1957b), "His only aim, and one which he never lost sight of, became to relieve the sufferings of mentally sick people" (p. 235). In 1908, Ferenczi met Sigmund Freud, and the two began a collaboration and a massive correspondence, now published in three volumes, that lasted 25 years until Ferenczi's death in 1933. The complexity of this relationship (Haynal, 1989b, 1992; Hoffer, 1996) includes mentorship (Freud generously helped Ferenczi get most of his early papers published), considerable mutual affection† (Freud at one point hoped that Ferenczi would marry his oldest daughter), traveling and vacation companions, "dependency"‡ (Ferenczi thought he

---

* For biographical information, I have depended on Berman (2004), Bókay (1998), Dupont (1994), Roazen (1975), and of course the Freud–Ferenczi correspondence.
† In Freud's words, it was an "intimate sharing of life, feelings, and interests" (Falzeder & Brabant, 2000).
‡ It would be easy to interpret their relationship in terms like those Bernard Brandchaft (see Chapter 7) called "systems of pathological accommodation," an intricate and hellish bargain in which the child or patient is forced to choose between the bond to the parent or analyst and the child's own self-development (Brandchaft, Doctors, & Sorter, 2010). See also Rudnytsky (2002) and Rudnytsky, Bókay, and Giampieri-Deutsch (1996). In the *Clinical Diary*, Ferenczi reproached Freud for not having analyzed his "negative transference." My own reading of the correspondence leads me to agree with Judith Vida (1997) in thinking that "dependency" does not adequately describe this complex relationship.

related to Freud as father-substitute, but it would be easy to argue that the dependency was bilateral), collaboration (strong evidence of mutual influence in the correspondence), domination and even exploitation by Freud, and ever-increasing divergence whose origins are evident in the correspondence from the beginning.* To complicate matters further, Freud, at Ferenczi's request, analyzed him for three brief periods in 1914 and 1916, a total of perhaps 6 weeks. Ferenczi, during one of Freud's periods of intense suffering from cancer, offered to travel to Vienna to analyze him, but Freud declined (appreciatively). In addition, as Vida (1997) noted, "Ferenczi employed his formidable talents to secure *Freud's voice* its central place in the psychoanalytic institutions that were just being developed" (p. 409, emphasis in original).

They diverged, primarily, over countertransference and over the centrality of trauma, two matters that encapsulate the whole problem of the attitude toward patients. Freud saw his own emotional reactions to patients as a nuisance factor, clouding his scientific lens and needing careful control. He wrote to Carl Jung in 1910 that he was beginning to understand the full importance of the rule "surmount counter-transference." To Ludwig Binswanger, whom Freud trusted more than he did Jung, he wrote,

> The problem of counter-transference, which you touch upon, is—technically—among the most intricate in psychoanalysis. Theoretically I believe it is much easier to solve. What we give to the patient should, however, be a spontaneous affect, but measured out consciously at all times, to a greater or lesser extent according to need. In certain circumstances a great deal, but never from one's own unconscious. I would look upon that as the formula. One must, therefore, always recognize one's counter-transference and

---

* It may be difficult for American readers to imagine how close Vienna and Budapest are and that it was easily possible for Ferenczi to attend the Wednesday evening meetings at Bergasse 19. In addition, both men spoke several languages, and their correspondence—with each other and with others—is peppered with expressions in English, French, Italian, and Latin. They wrote and spoke to each other in German, though Ferenczi's first language was Hungarian.

overcome it, for not till then is one free oneself. To give someone too little because one loves him too much is unfair to the patient and a technical error. This is all far from easy, and perhaps one has to be older for it, too. (Freud, Fichtner, & Binswanger, 2003, p. 160)

Ferenczi, by contrast, believed he needed to understand his own reactions and begged Freud to analyze him. He also, even when feeling most injured by Freud—as early as 1910*—urged Freud to consider his own emotional contribution to their interactions. But the profound mutuality that Ferenczi sought was not available with Freud. In the early 1920s he found Georg Groddeck, whose interest in what Winnicott would later call the "psyche-soma," and whose capacity for playfulness, gave Ferenczi a space for creativity less constrained than in his complex situation with Freud (Ferenczi, Fortune, & Groddeck, 2001; Rudnytsky, 2002).

In the last 10 years of his life (Haynal & Falzeder, 1993), Ferenczi, ever more determined to help his patients, experimented. His "active techniques" included setting rigid termination dates, forbidding certain activities, and so on, until he realized that these were no more helpful than Freud's "normal technique" of nongratification and indifference.† Indeed, in Axel Hoffer's (1991) words, "Ferenczi became aware that his active technique was the equivalent of harsh abuse of patients by an authoritarian figure, the unwitting reenactment of the original trauma at the hands of a tyrannical father" (p. 467). He then tried what he called the

---

* Repeatedly, Freud would invite Ferenczi to collaborate with him and then put him in his place. In the infamous Palermo incident of 1910, of which both later wrote, Freud had, as Ferenczi understood him, said that they would work together on the Schreber paper, but then Freud began to dictate it to him. Ferenczi stood up and asked, "This is what you mean by working together?" to which Freud responded, "So you want to take the whole thing?" There are many more examples in the correspondence where Ferenczi referred to his "father transference," but he also occasionally suggested that Freud consider whether he too was contributing something to their misunderstandings.
† Freud's German words that in English are usually rendered *neutrality* are *Neutralität* and *Indifferenz*.

"relaxation"* method (Ferenczi, 1930), attempting to make the patient as comfortable as possible, so that traumatic memories could return and be connected with the symptoms.

At the same time, from the time of his collaboration and break with Otto Rank in 1924–1925, Ferenczi was moving toward a form of psychoanalysis less modeled on the natural sciences—the world he and Freud had always shared—toward one centered on clinical practice, that is, a dialogic or hermeneutic psychoanalysis (Bókay, 1998). Indeed, impelled by his intense desire to understand and help his least "analyzable" patients, he stretched his practices and sometimes himself almost to the breaking point. Long before Gadamer would develop his dialogic hermeneutics as a philosophical phenomenology, Ferenczi developed a give-and-take clinical hermeneutics, in which the patient's meaning could always dispute the authority of the previously unchallenged analyst. Meanings emerged from clinical process, not from theory.

In his last years, chronicled in his *Clinical Diary* (Ferenczi & Dupont, 1988), he undertook his most difficult explorations in mutual analysis. His work with Elizabeth Severn (Fortune, 1993; Haynal, 1989b) and other severely traumatized patients in these years distanced him from Freud and thus created enormous personal strain for him. He had concluded that what had actually happened to children—especially including early sexual misuse—really mattered and, together with the indifference and obfuscation of adults, really was at the root of the worst psychological catastrophes. For Ferenczi, trauma (Greek for *injury*) always included two moments (Dupont, 1998) if it were to become pathogenic: the original shocking or repetitive abuse or neglect, followed by the disavowal, hypocrisy, and rejection both by the perpetrators and by others to whom the devastated child might have turned. In the words of Judit Mezaros (2010),

---

* Roazen understands *relaxation* here as referring to relaxation of the rigidity of the standard technique. Perhaps both meanings are present.

It was not a question of whether memories portray real events. He was asking what it was that turned an experience into a traumatic force for the subject … he placed the process of traumatization into a field of relations in which objective reality is colored by the relationship between the traumatized individual and the aggressor as well as by any number of other phenomena.* (p. 83)

Although in his early work Ferenczi had always attempted to keep his work within the Freudian framework, even producing critiques of those Freud came to ostracize, from the late 1920s he seemed to know he was going his own way. Collaborating with his patient Elizabeth Severn (the "R. N." of the *Clinical Diary*; Ferenczi & Dupont, 1988), he produced a complex and elaborated account of psychological trauma (Aron & Frankel, 1994). At the same time, just as his health declined from pernicious anemia at the end of his life, he produced papers that, even today, are decisive for our thinking about trauma and clinical process. A few months before his death, as he would normally do before presenting at a major congress, he read his "Confusion of Tongues" paper (1988) to Freud, giving his advocacy for the suffering child in the adult patient full voice (Vida, 1997). Freud walked away from him, having refused to shake his hand.

After his death, the psychoanalytic community, led by Ernest Jones but with the collusion of many others, suppressed Ferenczi's "Confusion of Tongues" paper until 1949, when Michael Balint is said to have persuaded Jones to allow its publication (Erwin, 2002). When Jones published the third volume of his Freud biography in 1956, he alleged that, as evidenced by his differences with Freud, Ferenczi had been insane in the years before his death. Many other sources dispute Jones's assertion as an attempt to discredit Ferenczi and either to keep his innovative thinking marginalized or to enhance Jones's own legacy in the history of psychoanalysis

---

* A similar account appears in intersubjective systems theory with its experiential-world-shattering, unmet by a "relational home" for the traumatic experience (Stolorow, 2007). We can agree with Haynal (1989a) that trauma is an economic concept—an injury that overwhelms the ego—only if we understand, as Ferenczi did, that this injury includes the relational context.

(Balint, 1958; Bonomi, 1998; Dupont, 1988; Roazen, 1975). Hoffer and Hoffer (1999) believe that Ferenczi did indeed suffer brief psychotic episodes as part of the pernicious anemia from which he died but that these in no way diminish the importance of his last writings. But also as Judit Dupont (1988) noted, "Those who get too close to the insane are always looked upon with suspicion" (p. 258). Carlo Bonomi (1999) has written an extensive and careful account of the entire controversy over Jones's allegations that place them in historical context. He believes, and I agree, that Ferenczi's challenge to the analyst's authority was too great for most even to consider until recently.

Paul Roazen, who wrote his masterful *Freud and His Followers* (1975) before either Ferenczi's *Clinical Diary* or the Freud–Ferenczi correspondence were available to us, did, however, have the opportunity to interview living people who had known Ferenczi and reported, "The faces of persons who knew Ferenczi still light up at the mention of his name" (p. 359). Even Jones knew it: "What we saw was the sunny, benevolent, inspiring leader and friend. ... With his open childlike nature, his internal difficulties, and his soaring fantasies, [Ferenczi] made a great appeal to Freud. He [Ferenczi] was in many ways a man after his own heart" (p. 359).

It is not surprising, therefore, that the rift between Ferenczi and Freud—even if never a full break—has been such a trauma for the psychoanalytic world (Balint, 1968), comparable to the loss of a parent. In this case, as in many families, the history is told as if the one parent had never existed. Anna Freud resisted publishing the correspondence, so that only now do we have the largest of Freud's bodies of informal and personal writing. On Ferenczi's side, he became the psychoanalytic family secret. Even now, even with the founding of the Ferenczi Center at the New School University in 2008, many analysts whose work clearly resembles his seem embarrassed to mention their kinship or indebtedness to him. It seems to me well past time for psychoanalysts and all humanistic psychotherapists to acknowledge our debts to him, without excessive idealizing, to see what we can still learn from him, and to draw strength from his courage.

FERENCZI'S OWN HERMENEUTICS

The story of Ferenczi's relationship with Freud could be told as one in which he moved from Freud's hermeneutics of suspicion to a "hermeneutics of trust" in the style of Hans-Georg Gadamer (Dostal, 1987). By the time we meet him in the texts we consider next, he has become a fully Gadamerian hermeneut, who listens to his patients, expecting to learn something. He has almost completely abandoned the hermeneutics of suspicion. But how did he reach this point? I suggest as a working hypothesis that finding himself openly met by Georg Groddeck (Ferenczi, Fortune, & Groddeck, 2001) allowed him to feel the real emotional pain of his patients with less evasion. Through embracing a hermeneutics of trauma, that is, by allowing the suffering of others to traumatize him (Lévinas, 1981), he began to trust the embodied voices of shattered people.

All the texts we consider here, with the exception of the first fragment, belong to his last three years, when he had privately withdrawn from his close collaboration with Freud and become a completely original voice in the history of psychoanalysis. The concept of trauma unites these texts, and none makes sense without it. For Ferenczi, as noted previously, trauma is both reality and experience. As Bowlby (1979) would later proclaim so firmly—and also find himself excluded from orthodox psychoanalysis for this view—what happens to children really matters to their development. Likewise, Ferenczi believed it crucial to take his patients seriously when they claimed to have been abused or otherwise mistreated, even when they asserted that *he* was mistreating or misunderstanding them.

At the same time, he fully shared our contemporary view of trauma as experience (Orange, 2011; Stolorow, 2007; Stolorow, Atwood, & Orange, 2002). The response of the surrounding others to the event is decisive for its development as psychological devastation that involves fragmentation, splitting of the psyche, and even, he thought, partial psychic death:

> Trauma is a process of dissolution that moves toward total dissolution, that is to say death. The body, the cruder part of the personality, withstands destructive processes longer, but unconsciousness and the fragmentation of the mind already are signs of the death of the more refined parts of the personality. Neurotics and psychotics, even if they are still halfway capable of fulfilling their functions as body and also partly as mind, should actually be considered to be unconsciously in a chronic death-agony. Analysis therefore has two tasks: (1) to expose this death-agony fully: (2) to let the patient feel that life is nevertheless worth living if there exist people like the helpful doctor, who is even prepared to sacrifice part of himself. (Ferenczi & Dupont, 1988, pp. 130–131)

In fact, he thought, the patient in treatment "must encounter enough compassion and sympathy that it seems worth his while to come back to life" (Ferenczi & Dupont, 1988, p. 40). Although this "helpful doctor" may sound grandiose, masochistic, or a candidate for imminent burnout, an alternative reading takes Ferenczi as saying, as Winnicott would later imply about his "regressed" patients and Fromm-Reichmann about schizophrenics, that such patients, as the condition for the possibility of hope, need to encounter someone like the "helpful doctor." Lévinasian "substitution," as we saw in Chapter 2, concerns the *possibility* of self-sacrifice for the suffering other, not its constant actuality.

Still, to read the late Ferenczi is to enter a hermeneutics of trauma. What does this imply? Primarily it shifts our focus *away from what is wrong with the patient*, that is, with pathology, *to what has happened to the patient to cause such extreme distress*. This shift in turn creates the needed transformation in the therapist's attitude that is the focus of most of the reflections in the *Clinical Diary*. Not until you stop analyzing my pathology, and start understanding what in you is obstructing your compassion,*

---

* Here, by the way, Peter Kravitz reminds me, lies a link to a Buddhist sensibility.

will you be able to help me, his patients told him over and over. Ferenczi's patients told him again and again that not until he recognized his own traumatic experience could he be on familiar terms with theirs and sincerely come to care for them. His work became a dialogic hermeneutics of trauma.

Clinicians may argue that their daily work is not so extreme, but we must remember that Ferenczi, like the others we consider in this book, devoted himself to those patients others considered "unanalyzable," hopeless cases. He was known as the analyst of last resort. It has been my experience that learning to understand those suffering from devastation, comparable to the world-collapse described by Jonathan Lear (2006), lights up everyday clinical work. The unnoticed suffering strangers become understandable and more accessible after we have worked with the despairing and the left-for-dead.

Let us therefore consider some uniquely Ferenczian themes that expressed his ability to see the suffering stranger/child in his adult patients, that is, his version of a hermeneutics of trust.

THE WISE BABY

Sometimes, the despairing turn up in very competent outward guises, so that their trauma does not immediately become visible. During the period of his closest collaboration with developmentalist Otto Rank, Ferenczi (1980) published for the first time his account of the dream of the clever baby:

> Not too seldom patients narrate to one dreams in which the newly born, quite young children, or babies in the cradle, appear, who are able to talk or write fluently, treat one to deep sayings, carry on intelligent conversations, deliver harangues, give learned explanations, and so on. I imagine that behind such dream-contents something typical is hidden ... the wish to become great and to excel over "the great" in wisdom and knowledge is only a reversal of the contrary situation of the child ... we should not forget that the young child is familiar with much knowledge, as a

matter of fact, that later becomes buried by the force of repression. (pp. 349–350)

Long before Ferenczi expanded on this theme in his last papers, he had noticed, possibly first in himself, how some precociously capable infants, toddlers, and young children have already become very intelligent caregivers, full of what today we might call "emotional intelligence" (Balint, 1957b; Goleman, 1995). Like the biblical scholar who uses the understanding of a strange passage, here a dream, to interpret the larger text, Ferenczi's "wise baby" became a kind of "portkey" (Rowling, 2000) into the understanding of patients traumatized by sexual violence, by the absence of the parental care that every child needs, and by the premature induction into weighty responsibilities for the emotional well-being of the adults who had injured and abandoned them. This early text, over the next 10 years of his clinical experimentation, evolved into two more elaborated versions.

> Many years ago I made a short communication on the relatively common occurrence of a typical dream: I called it the dream of the learned infant. I was referring to those dreams in which a newborn or very young infant in the cradle suddenly begins to talk and to give wise advice to its parents or other grown-ups. Now in one of my cases the intelligence of the unhappy child in the analytic phantasy behaved like a separate person whose duty it was to bring help with all speed to a child almost mortally wounded. "Quick, quick! what shall I do? They have wounded my child! There is no one to help! He is bleeding to death! He is scarcely breathing! I must bind up his wound myself. Now, child, take a deep breath or you will die. Now his heart has stopped beating! He is dying! He is dying!" (Ferenczi, 1931, pp. 476–477)

This second version of the wise baby dream clearly belongs already to the hermeneutics of trauma. Ferenczi has heard the voice and seen the face of the urgently calling child, almost mortally wounded, who though in a dissociated state, could then show him what had happened.

> The associations, which followed from the analysis of a dream, now ceased, and the patient was seized with an opisthotonus* and made movements as though to protect his abdomen. He was almost comatose, but I succeeded in establishing contact with him again and inducing him, with the help of the kind of encouragement and interrogation that I have described, to tell me about a sexual trauma of his early childhood. What I want to emphasize now is the light that this observation, and others like it, throw on the genesis of the narcissistic dissociation of the self. It really seems as though, under the stress of imminent danger, part of the self splits off and becomes a psychic institution which observed and desired to help the self, and that possibly this happens in early—even the very earliest—childhood. We all know that children who have suffered much morally or physically take on the appearance and mien of age and sagacity. They are prone to "mother" others also; obviously they thus extend to others the knowledge painfully acquired in dealing with their own sufferings, and they become kind and ready to help. It is, of course, not every such child who gets so far in mastering his own pain: many remain arrested in self-observation and hypochondria. (Ferenczi, 1931, p. 477)

Here we see Ferenczi the hermeneut at work in the clinical situation. Responding to a "wise baby" dream, he found himself with a patient in a body-memory with whom he worked to make contact. In conversation with the patient, he guessed that a self-split or "narcissistic dissociation" had occurred to create a helper for the child who was being assaulted, physically and psychologically. In this way this child becomes at once both extremely terrified and hypercapable. When we see in our practices patients who seem to alternate between these two possibilities, we ought perhaps to remember Ferenczi's clever baby.

As we will see next, he sometimes hypothesized that this helper child, the wise baby, could survive to become invested, even overinvested, in curing and relieving suffering—"a little psychiatrist"—while the rest of the original child either died or was relegated to preservation as an oddity (see discussion below

---

* "A condition of spasm of the muscles of the back, causing the head and lower limbs to bend backward and the trunk to arch forward" (*Merriam-Webster* online).

of the "teratoma" metaphor). Ferenczi's idea survives as the "parentified child" of contemporary talk and perhaps even as Alice Miller's (1979) "gifted child" whose life has been usurped by self-absorbed, self-serving, or violent parents. Indeed, it clearly occurred to Ferenczi that many wise babies survive to become psychotherapists, living out their own traumatic family history.*

Here is the third and final version from Ferenczi's (1949a) "Confusion of the Tongues":

> When subjected to a sexual attack, under the pressure of such traumatic urgency, the child can develop instantaneously all the emotions of mature adult and all the potential qualities dormant in him that normally belong to marriage, maternity and fatherhood. One is justified—in contradistinction to the familiar regression—to speak of a traumatic progression, of a precocious maturity. It is natural to compare this with the precocious maturity of the fruit that was injured by a bird or insect. Not only emotionally, but also intellectually, can the trauma bring to maturity a part of the person. I wish to remind you of the typical "dream of the wise baby" described by me several years ago in which a newly-born child or an infant begins to talk, in fact teaches wisdom to the entire family. The fear of the uninhibited, almost mad adult changes the child, so to speak, into a psychiatrist and, in order to become one and to defend himself against dangers coming from people without self-control, he must know how to identify himself completely with them. Indeed it is unbelievable how much we can still learn from our wise children, the neurotics. (p. 229)

Why do I say that "Ferenczi the hermeneut" noticed and understood the wise baby? The patients brought the text of the dream—as in the early biblical hermeneutics—to their analyst as analytic patients have always done. Ferenczi, already long convinced of mutual involvement in the analytic/therapeutic process and inclined toward dialogue, listened and heard in the open and

---

* Judith Vida (1996) provided a rich development of the wise baby idea and an illustrative clinical example.

trusting style that Gadamer would later theorize. The patient, accustomed to acceptance and support from his analyst, entered a state of traumatic memory in which the caregiver-child part of himself called on himself (and perhaps on Ferenczi) to give emergency care to the dying part of his child-self. Ferenczi participated not only in the emergency care but then in its joint understanding, exemplifying the use of hermeneutic understanding for the sake of responding to the suffering stranger. His clinical work, therefore, implies a belief that something of the injured child also may survive to be reunited with the adult "wise baby" if the analyst understands and cares sincerely enough.

Why could he do this when others of his era considered such patients "unanalyzable"? We can only guess. He seems to have understood, as others had not yet, that his own early traumatic experiences (sexual trauma, maternal coldness, loss of his father) had left him to be a clever baby, had already prepared him to care for others' sufferings. (He did not seem to have considered that being one of so many siblings could also have left him to fill in maternal functions.) He also seems to have tried to face his own wounds head-on, nonevasively, but could never find the analyst for himself that he was trying to be for others. After years of intense engagement with Freud in the creation of psychoanalytic theory, Freud's words to him "'patients are a rabble' ... patients only serve to provide us with a livelihood and material to learn from. We certainly cannot help them" (Ferenczi & Dupont, 1988, p. 93) convinced Ferenczi that their two attitudes toward psychoanalysis differed in basic ways. No matter what psychoanalytic critics might say, he had to search out ways to reach out to and understand the traumatized patient.

CONFUSION OF THE TONGUES BETWEEN THE ADULTS AND THE CHILD

And the Lord came down to see the city [Babel] and the tower ... and the Lord said, "Behold they are one people, and they have all one language; and this is only the beginning of what they will do; and nothing that they propose to do will now be impossible for them. Come, let us go down, and there confuse their language, that they may not understand."

—**Genesis 11:5–7,** *Revised Standard Version*

The source of the final dispute between Freud and Ferenczi concerned Freud's view that Ferenczi had, in his final paper—the Wiesbaden congress paper—simply returned to the trauma theory that Freud had abandoned 30 years earlier. According to Freud's original theory, hysterical symptoms encoded memories of early sexual seduction by caregivers, and the talking cure released the patient from the symptoms by decoding the memories. Freud had soon become convinced, of course, that most neuroses came from fantasized incest, that is, from the wished-for intimacies of the oedipal period, not from actual child molestation or other mistreatment of children. Ferenczi, on the other hand, wished above all to give credence to patients' tales of abuse—some of his adult patients had even told him they (and others they knew) had done such things to children—but knew that the effects were very complex and damaging and deserved to be studied and described. His account of what he called "traumatism"* elaborated a takeover of the child's entire being, a process Ferenczi named "identification with the aggressor."† The title of the paper itself refers to a double confusion: First, the adult confuses the child's desire for tender and affectionate interactions with an adultlike request for sexual relations, and second, the subsequent lies and denials confuse the child about what happened, whether anything happened, and whose initiative was involved. The child, now our patient, generally

---

* Both Ferenczi and Lévinas used the word *traumatism*, and neither, to my knowledge, defined it. It may stand for the way trauma spreads to include and freeze up more and more of life, including the people closely involved with a traumatized person, such as family members and analysts. It may also refer to the confusion not only of tongues but of temporality so that the traumatized feel strangely disoriented and "lose time."
† Ferenczi's concept has been the subject of a recent conversation (Berman, 2002; Bonomi, 2002; Frankel, 2002).

believes herself or himself absolutely to have been to blame, both for whatever occurred initially and for the continuing confusion and distress. Thus the patient, who was the child, has identified with the aggressor's version of the story and has taken on the guilt rejected by the perpetrator. Here are excerpts from this famous, long-suppressed* paper:

> A typical way in which incestuous seductions may occur is this: an adult and a child love each other, the child nursing the playful phantasy of taking the role of mother to the adult. This play may assume erotic forms but remains, nevertheless, on the level of tenderness. It is not so, however, with pathological adults, especially if they have been disturbed in their balance and self-control by some misfortune or by the use of intoxicating drugs. They mistake the play of children for the desires of a sexually mature person or even allow themselves—irrespective of any consequences—to be carried away. The real rape of girls who have hardly grown out of the age of infants, similar sexual acts of mature women with boys, and also enforced homosexual acts, are more frequent occurrences than has hitherto been assumed. (Ferenczi, 1949a, p. 227)

First we notice the intersubjective misunderstanding. The adult misinterprets the child's ordinary curiosity and the desire for playfulness and tenderness and responds with sexual passion, all the way to the rape of infants and children.[†]

> It is difficult to imagine the behavior and the emotions of children after such violence. One would expect the first impulse to be that of rejection, hatred, disgust and energetic refusal. "No, no, I do not want it, it is much too violent for me, it hurts, leave me alone," this or something similar would be the immediate reaction if it would not be paralyzed by enormous anxiety. These children feel physically and morally helpless, their personalities are not sufficiently consolidated in order to be able to protest, even if only in thought,

---

* Interested readers can find a detailed account of this suppression in Ferenczi and Dupont (1988) and Rachman (1997b).
† What Ferenczi seems not to have considered, possibly because his practice did not bring him such contacts, were violent abuses of children by strangers or other outsiders like clerics and teachers, children already emotionally abandoned by their families who then have nowhere to turn. Their tongues are also, but differently, confused.

for the overpowering force and authority of the adult makes them dumb and can rob them of their senses. (pp. 227–228)

The first reaction of traumatic shock and pain prevents protest, setting up the self-destruction Ferenczi named "identification with the aggressor."

> The same anxiety, however, if it reaches a certain maximum, compels them to subordinate themselves like automata to the will of the aggressor, to divine each one of his desires and to gratify these; completely oblivious of themselves they identify themselves with the aggressor. Through the identification, or let us say, introjection of the aggressor, he disappears as part of the external reality, and becomes intra- instead of extra-psychic; the intra-psychic is then subjected, in a dream-like state as is the traumatic trance, to the primary process, i.e. according to the pleasure principle it can be modified or changed by the use of positive or negative hallucinations. In any case the attack as a rigid external reality ceases to exist and in the traumatic trance the child succeeds in maintaining the previous situation of tenderness. (p. 228)

Again we see "identification with the aggressor," Ferenczi's description of the child's defensive self-loss in the face of devastating and overwhelming pain and confusion. He used the words "identification" and "introjection" almost interchangeably. As Frankel (2002) noted, Anna Freud (1967) later gave this defense the sense it has for most people: becoming an aggressor oneself so that one no longer has to feel oneself a victim. She thus appealed to the common observation that bullied children often turn to beat down children smaller or otherwise more vulnerable than themselves. Ferenczi, on the contrary, had been describing the experience of the traumatized child who felt—partly because the adult afterward said so—that he or she had wanted or created the incest or provoked the violence or abandonment. It has been my own observation that even a child unwanted from before birth, as Ferenczi (1929) too had noted, often feels that there is something repulsive or defective about himself or herself that makes the rejection reasonable.

Identification with the aggressor, in the Ferenczian sense, describes the everyday clinical experience of patients who are completely convinced that because others have rejected them, they truly belong outside the human community. Possibly we find here the earliest roots of the horrible shame so well described by Morrison (1987, 1999) and others (Gump, 2000; Kilborne, 1999; Lansky, 1994; Orange, 2008b). From the outset we have identified with the others who have felt themselves, and then treated us, as burdens, as intrusions, as nuisances, as toys to be used and discarded, as useful adjuncts, as worthless, lazy, selfish, good-for-nothing, even as evil, or, in the words of Ferenczi, as "little psychiatrists," and so we have developed our sense of ourselves. Often we grow up feeling ourselves to be a confused mixture of these humiliated identifications, and so we arrive, defeated and despairing, feeling guilty for what others have done "as if I raped myself," at the therapist's door. As Brandchaft's similar, though not identical, account will also show, the aggressor's agenda has taken over the whole being of the child who becomes our patient. This pervasive damage may or may not be immediately evident, but a therapist attuned to the depths of shame and bewilderment may begin to sense the traumatism. "The most important change, produced in the mind of the child by the anxiety-fear-ridden identification with the adult partner, is the introjection of the guilt feelings of the adult which makes hitherto harmless play appear as a punishable offence" (Ferenczi, 1949a, p. 228).

Of course, only with difficulty does the patient—or a therapist with a similar history, perhaps—connect this confusion and shame with its origins, because our tongues can also be confused in this very identification with the aggressor. In Ferenczi's (1949a) words,

> When the child recovers from such an attack, he feels enormously confused, in fact, split—innocent and culpable at the same time—and his confidence in the testimony of his own senses is broken. Moreover, the harsh behavior of the adult partner tormented and made angry by his remorse renders the child still more conscious

of his own guilt and still more ashamed. Almost always the perpetrator behaves as though nothing had happened, and consoles himself with the thought: "Oh, it is only a child, he does not know anything, he will forget it all." (pp. 228–229)

The perpetrator is both right and wrong. The adult patient does not remember the origins of his or her suffering in any way that is now useful. Instead one carries the suffering in embodied memory, psychosomatically, as Ferenczi learned from his collaboration with Georg Groddeck. Or one lives dissociated: "A helpless child is mistreated, for example through hunger. What happens when the suffering increases and exceeds the small person's power of comprehension? Colloquial usage describes what follows by the expression 'the child comes to *be beside itself*'" (Ferenczi & Dupont, 1988, p. 32). In the clinical situation, clinicians may notice that such patients speak of "the baby" or "the child" without awareness that they are speaking as if of someone else.

The confusion of tongues also returns us to the theme of the wise baby. Not only sexually abused children have their tongues confused, though these most violently do:

> In addition to passionate love and passionate punishment there is a third method of helplessly binding a child to an adult. This is the terrorism of suffering. Children have the compulsion to put to rights all disorder in the family, to burden, so to speak, their own tender shoulders with the load of all the others; of course this is not only out of pure altruism, but is in order to be able to enjoy again the lost rest and the care and attention accompanying it. A mother complaining of her constant miseries can create a nurse for life out of her child, i.e. a real mother substitute, neglecting the true interests of the child. (Ferenczi, 1949a, p. 229)

Though, as Haynal (1989) noted, Ferenczi was fascinated by catastrophe theories in geology and paleontology, his theory of psychological trauma included both catastrophes like sexual attacks on children and the continual misuse, neglect, exploitation, and misattunement that Khan (1963) would later name "cumulative trauma" and Bernard Brandchaft (2007) would name "systems of pathological accommodation" (see Chapter 7). This "terrorism of suffering" was fully capable of creating a wise baby, admired all around but really living outside itself and much more precariously organized and lost to itself than anyone thinks until Humpty Dumpty—who has sat, even if unwittingly, on the wall between "normality" and catastrophe for a lifetime—has a great fall (i.e., meets major retraumatization and perhaps breaks down).

It may be that such a wise baby becomes the "apparently normal personality" of the highest functioning people described by the trauma theorists of today (Hart, Nijenhuis, & Steele, 2006), whose embodied and emotional memories remain dissociated and largely unavailable to them. Developmental or relational trauma—whether abuse, neglect, usurpation, or some combination—may transform the child just as Ferenczi described long ago. Only when the system crashes, or when the barely surviving person meets a clinician prepared with the hermeneutics of trust, can the work of healing such fragmentation begin. Such patients need, Ferenczi believed, all the advantages of a normal nursery. They have never been allowed to be children, with the needs and dependency of children. Both Michael Balint (1968) and Donald Winnicott (1955) would call these needs regressive, but all three understood that many of these attachment needs had never been met and that the going-back was not to a refinding but to a desperate hope of finding the needed "something" for the first time. "The man abandoned by all the gods," Ferenczi (1949b) thought, might at the last moment find himself in his traumatic struggle

> no longer alone. Although we cannot offer him everything which he as a child should have had, the mere fact that we can or may be helpful to him gives the necessary impetus towards a new life in which the pages of the irretrievable are closed and where the first step will be made towards acquiescence in what life yet can offer instead of throwing away what may still be put to good use. (p. 234)

TERATOMA AND SPLITTING

We next consider some Ferenczian descriptions of the damage that very early and extreme trauma wreaks on the psyche.

> It is no mere poetic license to compare the mind of the neurotic to a double malformation, something like the so-called teratoma which harbors in a hidden part of its body fragments of a twin-being which has never developed. No reasonable person would refuse to surrender such a teratoma to the surgeon's knife, if the existence of the whole individual were threatened. ... I can picture cases of neurosis, in fact I have often met with them in which (possibly as a result of unusually profound shocks in infancy) the greater part of the personality becomes, as it were, a teratoma, the task of adaptation to reality being shouldered by the fragment of personality which has been spared. Such persons have actually remained almost entirely at the child-level, and for them the usual methods of analytical therapy are not enough. What such neurotics need is really to be adopted and to partake for the first time in their lives of the advantages of a normal nursery. (Ferenczi, 1930, pp. 441–442)

What is *teratoma*?* Stanton believes that teratoma remained a powerful but little developed metaphor for traumatic process, which he thought can leave behind a kind of "underdeveloped embryonic twin" (Stanton, 1991, p. 336), leaving the fragment that remains to live as if it were whole, under great strain.† Insofar as the trauma survivor is aware of the very young twin, it seems to him or her ugly and shameful—as the word *teratoma* suggests—and something to be rid of. In my experience, these traumatized patients apologize to me constantly, feeling what they see as their shameful and disgusting neediness as a terrible burden that no one should have to bear. They often tell me that their child-self is

---

* *Teratoma* is Greek for "monster," a medical term for "a unique form of tumor which contains all three of the germ layers of the developing embryo: it has skin and nervous tissue from the ectoderm, intestinal and glandular epithelium from the endoderm, and fibrous tissue, bone, and muscle from the mesoderm" (Rudnytsky et al., 1996; Stanton, 1991).

† Judith Vida (2001), on the contrary, thinks that Ferenczi saw the teratoma as an effect, not as the traumatic process itself.

already dead or should be surgically excised like a tumor because it causes only trouble.

Although aspects of Ferenczi's trauma work appear in much everyday clinical work and apply to adult trauma as well,* *teratoma* points to the damage wreaked by physical, emotional, and sexual violence to infants and small children, long before they can tell a story about it. Each of the clinical hermeneuts we study in this book perceived this devastation, recognized that orthodox psychoanalysis could not address it, and tried to find a response without leaving the psychoanalytic world completely.

Leonard Shengold (1979), who acknowledged his indebtedness to Ferenczi in his works on soul murder, explained the necessity for such splitting off:

> The child who is tormented by a parent must frequently call on that same parent for help and rescue … if the very parent who abuses and is experienced as bad must be turned to for relief of the distress that parent has caused, then the child must break with what he has experienced and must, out of desperate need, register the parent—delusionally—as good. Only the mental image of a good parent can help the child deal with the terrifying intensity of fear and rage which is the effect of the tormenting experiences … this is a mind-splitting or a mind-fragmenting operation. (p. 539)

Ferenczi saw these patients as in need of a normal nursery. What does this mean? Once again we see the compassionate effect of a hermeneutics of trauma and trust:

> The love and strength of the analyst, assuming that trust in him goes deep enough and is great enough, have nearly the same effect as the embrace of a loving mother and a protective father. The help offered by the mother's lap and strong embrace permits complete relaxation, even after a shattering trauma, so that the shattered person's own powers, undisturbed by the external tasks of precautions or defense, can devote themselves in an unsplintered way to the internal task of repairing the function-impairment

---

* For a description and treatment of adult trauma, see Boulanger (2002), and for an existential phenomenological account, see Stolorow (2007).

caused by the unexpected penetration. (Ferenczi & Dupont, 1988, pp. 68–69)

The analyst, according to Ferenczi, becomes a kind of papoose board or supportive splint for a badly fragmented person until enough healing can occur, especially through processes of mutual engagement in the unconfusion of tongues, past and present, to allow for more unbinding. This function, similar though not identical to the "holding environment"—which Winnicott saw as necessary for normal development—is additionally crucial because of the way Ferenczi understood what happens psychologically to a severely traumatized person:

> From the moment when bitter experience teaches us to lose faith in the benevolence of the environment, a permanent split in the personality occurs. The split-off part sets itself up as a guard against dangers, mainly on the surface (skin and sense organs), and the attention of this guard is almost exclusively directed toward the outside. It is concerned only with danger, that is to say, with the objects in the environment, which can all become dangerous. Thus the splitting of the world, which previously gave the impression of homogeneity, into subjective and objective psychic systems; each has its own way of remembering, of which only the objective system is actually completely conscious. … Only in sleep do we succeed, by means of certain external arrangements (creation of a secure situation by closing windows and doors, by wrapping ourselves in protective, warm bedclothes), in calling off this guard. (Ferenczi & Dupont, 1988, p. 69)

Here Ferenczi produces a radical alternative to the Freudian understanding of defense, a central part of the hermeneutics of suspicion. Once we understand the shattered person as desperately attempting to hold and protect the remaining fragments and shards, we develop a different hermeneutic, a way of hearing resistance and defense as almost heroic (again, more when we come to Kohut and Brandchaft).

ANALYTIC ATTITUDE

If a therapist, protecting her or his own emotional vulnerability,* meets such a patient with traditionally "neutral" and distant analytic attitudes, there is, Ferenczi learned, no hope. "The [usual] analytic technique creates transference, but then withdraws, wounding the patient without giving him a chance to protest or to go away; hence interminable fixation on the analysis while the conflict remains unconscious" (Ferenczi & Dupont, 1988, p. 210). Ferenczi asked a different question: How must an analyst or therapist meet such a patient, devastated by earlier or later mistreatment?

> If the patient notices that I feel real compassion for her and that I am eagerly determined to search for the causes of her suffering, she then suddenly not only becomes capable of giving a dramatic account of the events but also can talk to me about them. The congenial atmosphere thus enables her to project the traumata into the past and communicate them as memories. A contrast to the environment surrounding the traumatic situation—that is, sympathy, trust—mutual trust—must first be created before a new footing can be established: memory instead of repetition. Free association by itself, without these new foundations for an atmosphere of trust, will thus bring no real healing. The doctor must really be involved in the case, heart and soul, or honestly admit it when he is not, in total contrast with the behavior of adults toward children. (Ferenczi & Dupont, 1988, pp. 169–170)

Here we encounter Ferenczi's version of the central thesis of this book, developed in two previous chapters: Meeting the patient with attitudes formed by the hermeneutics of trust changes what becomes available for understanding. Suspicion may unmask but cannot heal.

> If the patient really feels that we will in fact take care of him, that we take his infantile need for help seriously (and one cannot offer a helpless child, which is what most patients are, mere

---

* Freud (1912) knew well that his "surgical" recommendations were designed not only to protect the reputation of psychoanalysis but also for this purpose: "This emotional coldness ... creates for the doctor a desirable protection for his own emotional life" (p. 115).

theories when it is in terrible pain), then we shall be able to induce the patient to look back into the past without terror. (Ferenczi & Dupont, 1988, p. 210)

The courage comes because the patient, still injured and terrified but no longer completely alone, comes to have a sense that perhaps she or he will not be left to perish, to die alone.

> It helps the analysis when the analyst is able, with almost inexhaustible patience, understanding, goodwill and kindliness, to meet the patient as far as possible. By so doing he lays up a reserve by means of which he can fight out the conflicts which are inevitable sooner or later, with a prospect of reconciliation. The patient will then feel the contrast between our behavior and that which he experienced in his real family and, knowing himself safe from the repetition of such situations, he has the courage to let himself sink down into a reproduction of the painful past. (Ferenczi, 1931, pp. 473–474)

Only when a therapist offers such a participatory and supportive understanding (the psychoanalytic witness; Orange, 1995; Poland, 2000) does the patient often fully realize the depth and extent of the injury, denial, and abandonment.

> In contrast to our own procedure, we then learn of the ill-advised and inappropriate actions and reactions of adults in the patient's childhood in the presence of the effects of traumatic shocks. Probably the worst way of dealing with such situations is that of denying their existence, of asserting that nothing has happened and that nothing is hurting the child. Sometimes he is actually beaten or scolded when he manifests traumatic paralysis of thought and motion. These are the kinds of treatment which make the trauma pathogenic. One gets the impression that children get over even severe shocks without amnesia or neurotic consequences, if the mother is at hand with understanding and tenderness and (what is most rare) with complete sincerity. (Ferenczi, 1931, p. 479)

At the same time, Ferenczi came to realize that if kindness and warmth were indispensible, they did not suffice. The analyst, with all her own frailties, with all the limitations resulting from her own emotional history, would surely harm the patient and be justly reproached:

> It is an unavoidable task for the analyst: although he may behave as he will, he may take kindness and relaxation as far as he possibly can, the time will come when he will have to repeat with his own hands the act of murder previously perpetrated against the patient. In contrast to the original murder, however, he is not allowed to deny his guilt.* (Ferenczi & Dupont, 1988, p. 52)

That we will inevitably retraumatize—"murder," he said—our patients, even when we have become capable of loving them, should make us humble. We remain finite beings, and no amount of elasticity (Ferenczi, 1930), wisdom, and compassion will give us enough time or endurance to make up to our patients (or to their significant others) for the crimes they have endured. Instead, we must acknowledge *our* crimes and misdemeanors, as kindly as possible; we must admit how little we understand, we must confess our exhaustion and frustration. We must accept responsibility for our current contribution to our patients' suffering (Vida, 1993). We must be sincere.

Nor should we expect (cf. Rudnytsky, 2002) that one episode of honesty and humility will be enough for someone who has learned to trust no one:

> It does not seem to suffice to make a general confession and to receive general absolution; patients want to see all the sufferings that we caused them corrected one by one, to punish us for them, and then to wait until we no longer react with defiance or by taking offense, but with insight, regret, indeed with loving sympathy. (Ferenczi & Dupont, 1988, p. 209)

In other words, an offhand "Yes, I make mistakes" or even "You are right, I shouldn't have done that" does not restore trust. A genuine apology acknowledges both the harm done to the other and sometimes even our less-than-generous motivation. It expresses

---

* This aspect of Ferenczi's work resonates with the contemporary American relational school's emphasis on enactment. See, for example, Aron and Harris (1993) and Harris and Aron (1997).

genuine sorrow. Sometimes it is necessary to say that I don't know exactly why I did or did not say something and that I will think it over and get back to you. If it turns out that I was actually being selfish, self-absorbed, or retaliatory, I may have to say so. If I was truly preoccupied and elsewhere, I may have to say so. Whatever the case, in Ferenczi's view the honesty demanded of patients in analysis required a matching sincerity on the analyst's side. He thus placed himself at risk, "without any insurance" (Haynal, 1993, p. 199), to an extent unthinkable among proponents of "standard technique." When our patients correct us, he said, "the analyst must swallow a good deal and he must learn to renounce his authority as an omniscient being" (Ferenczi, 1949b, p. 242). He had to acknowledge and accept having caused additional suffering to his patient and at the same time restore the comfort and hope needed to go on.

But this is not enough either. We have to change our way of being with the patient from the inside out. We have to find a way to love this patient. For Ferenczi, deprived of a good-enough analyst for himself, this meant engaging in his ultimately disappointing but informative experiments in mutual analysis.

MUTUALITY

Detractors have become so distracted by Ferenczi's experiments in mutual analysis—motivated, they claim with Freud, by Ferenczi's allegedly neurotic "*furor sanandi*" (passion to cure)*—that they miss his central message. To reach our most devastated patients, he believed, we must allow ourselves to be known, criticized, and changed by them—a massive challenge to the authoritarian orthodoxies in psychoanalysis and other forms of psychotherapy. Eleanor Roosevelt famously said that understanding was a two-way street, and so, Ferenczi taught us, is psychoanalysis. Today large groups in the psychoanalytic world are exploring this

---

* A welcome rehabilitation of therapeutic passion appears in Hoffman (2009b).

message: relational psychoanalysts, relational self psychologists, and intersubjective systems theorists. Outside psychoanalysis, a dialogic and relational approach is growing in the worlds of humanistic psychotherapies such as gestalt therapies (Hycner & Jacobs, 1995; Staemmler, 2009). But Ferenczi's own words, admittedly less theoretically developed because original in his time, still challenge us to live up to our fine theories: "One could almost say that the more weaknesses an analyst has, which lead to greater or lesser mistakes and errors but which are then uncovered and treated in the course of mutual analysis, the more likely the analysis is to rest on profound and realistic foundations" (Ferenczi & Dupont, 1988, p. 15).

Today's emphases on mutuality and intersubjectivity owe a profound debt to Ferenczi's willingness to place himself continually at risk on many levels but always, of course, for the sake of the sufferings of the traumatized. This attitude drove Ferenczi to his experiments with mutuality and convinced him that only together can we enter the path toward healing and reintegration. In the evocative words of Vida and Molad (2004),

> Being traumatized ... is the experience of facing annihilation. Reliving a trauma takes us back inside the experience with no sense of how it's going to end. There is no as-if, and no sense of the person one is in the present that travels into the reliving ... in the community of empty mouths communication can take place, with the exercise of personal responsibility, and in fact, *a transformational embrace* of mutual trauma is a possibility. (pp. 346–347)

They suggested that working in a Ferenczian spirit means working in the dark at times, embracing the risks of mutual retraumatization (Jaenicke, 2008), witnessing the other's suffering, and making and finding such a wholehearted psychoanalysis as a way of life. Antal Bókay (1998) eloquently expressed the effect that Ferenczi's shift to the hermeneutics of trust makes in our clinical life. In contrast to the "decent profession" of methodical and more distant psychoanalysis, Ferenczi's psychoanalysis involves free and mutual self-creation in which the participants are magicians, lovers, and true friends. Subjective existence and recovery take place in language. ... The dialogue in question is a real one: *we do not talk about our inner meaning using conversation as an instrument, but rather we exist in it.* (p. 196, emphasis added)

Gadamer could not have said it better.

In the end, Ferenczi's experiments, and his experience of the hazards of full mutual analysis for his other patients, led him to the conclusion: "Mutual analysis: only a last resort!" (Ferenczi & Dupont, 1988, p. 115). What can we conclude from his conclusion? He drew back, in the end, I believe, not from fear of his own inflated grandiosity or burnout. He believed that the dangers of grandiosity lay more on the side of holding a hypocritical and distantly authoritarian, theory-loaded analytic role. Allowing oneself to be constantly criticized, and seeking to meet the patient's needs, did not seem to him grandiose. Nor did he fear burnout, any more than did Winnicott (oh god, let me live until I die!). To discover what could help the most devastated, he would easily give his own life, it seems to me.* What turned him away from mutual analysis was the old medical adage "do no harm." He quickly found that the complexity of his and his patients' relationships made mutual analysis too costly for too many people, and he had to abandon it in the literal sense. What he learned from it, however, has been teaching psychoanalysis and psychotherapy about mutuality, intersubjectivity, and sincerity ever since.

CLINICAL HERMENEUTICS

It is possible to identify several humanistic clinical attitudes—surely not rules—as typically Ferenczian.

---

* We also need to remember that the pernicious anemia, from which he died, easily yields today to treatment with vitamin B_{12}.

The Patient's Needs Require the Analyst's Full Sincerity and Tact

In Balint's (1957a) paraphrase, "Ferenczi has shown us how we have to watch every tone, every movement, every gesture, so that only true sincerity should lead us and not the 'professional hypocrisy' which reduces the patient to silence" (p. 240).* We may note here that it is not a question of the "authenticity" so prized in contemporary psychoanalysis but rather, as Ferenczi repeatedly emphasized in his last years, that we had to find a way to transform any pretense of caring for our patient into something genuine. Until we could do this, we had better not pretend.

The tact and timing—some might say "strategy"—always valued in clinical work—does not disappear in this account. To wait for the opportune moment to raise a question can simply be a matter of developmental sensitivity, as both Ferenczi and Winnicott would agree. But anything phony will prevent the needed safety within which all the terrors can come out and be grappled with together.

Be Ready to Experiment

Ferenczi, ever a fallibilist (Orange, 1995), held his own ideas and those of others lightly. He, in Balint's (1957b) words, "never forgot that psychoanalysis was really discovered by a patient, Miss Anna O., and the merit of the physician, Dr. Breuer, lay in the very fact that he was always ready to accept his patient's guidance and to learn from her the new method of healing" (p. 238). Later, when Ferenczi stumbled in his own work, he took it as a sign that he himself needed further analysis. In his view, "If a patient is willing to continue the analysis and work still does not proceed, then it is the physician and his method that are at fault" (p. 238). In much the same spirit, a Gadamerian hermeneut expects always to be questioned by the other with whom we seek understanding.

---

* Balint had been Ferenczi's patient in the 1920s and was later his colleague, friend, and literary executor.

Be Ready to Acknowledge Mistakes and Negative Attitudes Toward the Patient

Again, in Balint's (1957a) words,

> He shrank from no sacrifice if, in the opinion of a patient, the treatment failed to progress because of his [Ferenczi's] personal peculiarities. He revised his words, his usual modes of expression, his gestures, even the pitch of his voice, if his patients criticized them; and he was always prepared, at whatever cost to himself, to examine the limits of his sincerity. He did not allow himself a single false or even a vacant tone in a patient's presence. (pp. 238–239)

Assume the Patient Is Wounded and Confused, Not Hostile

This forms a crucial premise of any therapeutics informed by a hermeneutics of trust and obviously contrasts with all forms of psychoanalysis and psychotherapy that assume aggressive motivations as psychological bedrock.

Assume That Defenses Serve Survival Needs

For example, "an important source of masochism: pain [may be] the alleviation of other greater pains" (Ferenczi & Dupont, 1988, p. 23). We will pursue this idea further in chapters on Heinz Kohut and Bernard Brandchaft.

Assume That the Patient Is Our Partner in the Search for Meaning

In the words of Vida and Molad (2004), "The elaboration of Ferenczi's ideas leads to a radically different conceptualization of the therapeutic encounter" (p. 339), in which the analyst no longer simply decodes the patient's unconscious meanings.

Finally, Ferenczi concluded, we need not choose between understanding and kindness. A few months before his death, reflecting on the long work with the most fragmented of his patients, he wrote,

> In addition to the capacity to integrate the fragments intellectually, there must also be kindness, as this alone makes the integration permanent. Analysis on its own is intellectual anatomical dissection. A child cannot be healed with understanding alone. It must be helped first in real terms and then with comfort and the awakening of hope. ... Kindness alone would not help much either, but only both together. (Ferenczi & Dupont, 1988, p. 207)

What Ferenczi had done, in short, was to place healing, not theory, in the center of psychoanalysis. Practice gave meaning to theory "rather than being merely its byproduct" (Bókay, 1998, p. 194). This practice involved a hermeneutics of trust that included treating patients with humanity and compassion. A Ferenczian hermeneutic psychoanalysis, Bókay continued, "is not a profession but a *way of life*, a self-creation through dialogue" (p. 194).

Perhaps poet Attila Jozsef,* the greatest Hungarian poet and contemporary of Ferenczi, said it best:

> You have made me the child again
> without a trace of thirty years of pain.
> I cannot move away, whatever I do
> it is to you I am drawn, despite myself.
> I have slept on the threshold
> far from a mother's arms
> hiding within myself, insane.
> Above, a vacant heaven;
> O sleep! it's at your door that I am knocking.
> There are those who weep in silence
> Yet seem hard like me,
> Look: my love for you is of such strength
> That I can love myself, with you.

---

* I owe this to Haynal (1989a).

A TALE OF TWO FERENCZIS

It seems to me that in contemporary psychoanalysis, in the years since the *Clinical Diary* and all three volumes of the Freud–Ferenczi correspondence have become available, we have come to have two versions of Ferenczi, almost another traumatic split in our memory of him.* First, we have the Ferenczi of mutual analysis, who told his patients what he could not bear about them and even more what his own failures were, the paradigm of mutuality and confrontation and egalitarianism and playing by ear. But we also have the maternal Ferenczi, generous and tender and compassionate, convinced that his patients' suffering and terror required an asymmetrical analytic relationship. His hermeneutics of trauma and trust had led him to believe his patients had actually suffered abuse and abandonment that needed more than a distant, intellectual knowledge. This second Ferenczi inspires those who believe that confrontation and frankness do not suffice but instead are probing to describe something like "analytic love" (Shaw, 2003). This second voice often gets lost in tales of what the patient is doing to the analyst. In my reading, throughout the *Clinical Diary*, Ferenczi alternated between these two attitudes as if he were fighting his own battle between them. He experimented with mutual analysis and came to value mutuality and sincerity so much, just because he came to understand them as the absolutely necessary conditions for the possibility of sustaining the maternal attitude. When he felt his own compassion breaking down or, worse yet, when his patients felt it breaking down, the two grown-ups had to explore together what kinds of evasions or dissociations, on both parts, might be interfering with healing the completely devastated child/adult who had entrusted a raped and shattered soul to this analyst. In these moments we need, he said, "the humble admission, in front of the patient, of one's own weaknesses and traumatic experiences and disillusionments, which

---

* Something similar may be happening with Winnicott.

abolishes completely that distancing by inferiority which would otherwise be maintained" (Ferenczi & Dupont, 1988, p. 65).

Note that this practice does not require a full-on mutual analysis; it *does* require the transformation in attitude that supported Ferenczi's clinical experiments. He continued,

> Should it even occur, as it does occasionally to me, that experiencing another's and my own suffering brings a tear to my eye (and one should not conceal this emotion from the patient), then the tears of doctor and of patient mingle in a sublimated communion, which perhaps finds its analogy only in the mother–child relationship. And this is the healing agent. (Ferenczi & Dupont, 1988, p. 65)

In a genuinely Lévinasian spirit, Ferenczi cared enough for the face of the suffering other to develop a hermeneutics of trust. Like others who followed this path, he paid a high price in rejection and misunderstanding.

So let us consider briefly Ferenczi's courage. With fear and trembling, but also with increasing confidence, he emerged from Freud's shadow to open himself to the face of his suffering patients who called to him, "Don't let me perish helplessly!" Where in our training are we taught to hear this call or to respond if we are able to hear it? Suppose it comes in a form previously unrecognized? Ferenczi refused to retreat to the familiar (Borgogno, 2004) and instead allowed his patients to lead him into the darkest, ugliest regions of human cruelty perpetrated on children and its devastating aftermath. His "child analysis in the analysis of adults" (Ferenczi, 1931) prefigured the work of Winnicott and left him vulnerable not only to rejection by Freud and slander by Jones but to oblivion until recent years. The wise baby grew up to leave psychotherapists the gift of his commitment and courage.

For the Lévinasian ethic, this path of commitment remains a radical path that we may not evade, unless we are willing to abandon our patients as they have already been abandoned. We may today know something more about mitigating "compassion fatigue" and "vicarious trauma" (Courtois & Ford, 2009) than Ferenczi knew. What he knew was that meeting each devastated patient would require a level of involvement and willingness to change that we could not imagine in advance.

"AND WE SHALL BE CHANGED"

"The trumpet shall sound," proclaims the basso in G. F. Händel's famous aria, "And we shall be changed."* In psychoanalysis, we may not hear the trumpet of theological expectation, but if we surrender ourselves to the intersubjective complexity into which Ferenczi invites and challenges us, we will be profoundly changed. According to contemporary intersubjectivist Chris Jaenicke (2011), in psychoanalytic treatment "a meeting of subjective worlds occurs in which we are called upon to partially reorganize our basic organizing principles ... unless we are able to meet this challenge, to embrace this depth of involvement, the therapy will not have a lasting effect. To change, we have to let ourselves be changed" (p. 14). The question, he said, that our patients pose to us "is whether we are willing to go to the bottom with them" (p. 29). Though in the end Ferenczi understood that literal mutual analysis—the result of his own unsuccessful analysis with Freud—had to fail, he remained committed to the idea that any fully engaged analysis must transform both people. To explain the "therapeutic action" in intersubjective systems (Orange, Atwood, & Stolorow, 1997; Stolorow et al., 2002) or relational terms (Mitchell, 2000a), I must describe what both parties bring to the field, how complex and interdependent are the processes of mutual influence and asymmetric (Lévinasian) role responsibility. I must relate how both of us have been changed by each other and by the work/play/struggle we have done together.

By you who walk through my door in the next hour with your unique need to be met and embraced, despite whatever I may

---

* This concluding section is adapted from my Foreword to Jaenicke (2011).

bring that hinders or complicates my compassion, I am humbled and changed. In the face of your grief so immense that it seems a dying of sorrow right here before me, I am transformed in ways for which I have no words. In the face of your challenge not to ignore your despair by taking up easier problems, I am changed. In the face of your apparent wealth and privilege that reawakens my rotten shame, I am changed. In the face of your history of violence and abandonment that reminds me of my own degradation but also that we share a common humanity, I am changed. In the face of your soul murder by parents who unleashed their hatred and cruelty upon you, and who even now thwart all my capacity and desire to comfort and protect, I am humbled. In the face of your need and desire, child and adult, to be uniquely loved and cherished, and my own complex needs to love and to cherish as well as to be loved, I am challenged and changed. As a result of our personal "participation in the suffering of the patient" (Jaenicke), "we shall be changed" (Händel). Understanding all this, I owe first to my patients and second to Ferenczi.

4
Frieda Fromm-Reichmann
Incommunicable Loneliness

> *Frieda single-handedly contributed more than any other individual to encourage all of the western world to apply psychotherapy to schizophrenics.*
>
> **—Alberta Szalita**

Frieda Fromm-Reichmann, a petite immigrant from Nazi Germany, made an immense contribution to a distinctively American therapeutic sensibility. Her straightforward way of speaking of clinical process, combined with her personal dedication to doing whatever it might take to reach the schizophrenic patient in her care, placed her outside the mainstream of the psychoanalytic establishment.* Nevertheless, she constantly credited Freud with having made the pivotal step that made understanding the suffering of the mentally ill possible. "Did you ever realize," she often asked her students,

---

* Klaus Hoffmann (1998) rightly remarked on her ecumenism: "Fromm-Reichmann not only became a member of the German Psychoanalytic Society, she also joined the General Medical Society for Psychotherapy, the members of which were mainly of physicians, quite a few of them being very critical towards psychoanalysis. The other way round, the German Psychoanalytic Society remained very skeptical towards the Society of Psychotherapy. Fromm-Reichmann was very ecumenical—as later in the United States where she was a member of the American Psychoanalytic Association as well as the William Alanson White Institute!" (p. 92).

what an ingenious deed of Freud's it was to make the demand to tell everything that comes into your mind? Do you realize what enormous courage it took to ask that from people who live within our culture which is so full of suppression and repression, and where nearly everybody lives under the continual strain of not telling undisguised what comes into his mind from fear of getting hostile reactions from his surroundings? (Hornstein, 2000, pp. 45–46)

Already we can hear her distinctive voice, clear about what she accepted from tradition, as she would also be about her differences. In her own work,

> The patient is asked neither to lie down nor to give free associations; both requests make no sense to [psychotics]. He should feel free to sit, lie on the floor, walk around, use any available chair, lie or sit on the couch. ... If the patient feels that an hour of mutual friendly silence serves his purpose, he is welcome to remain silent. ... Nothing matters except that the analyst permit the patient to feel comfortable and secure enough to give up his defensive narcissistic isolation and to use the physician for resuming contact with the world. (Fromm-Reichmann, 1959, p. 123)

She insisted that we had to listen very closely, with more awareness of our own struggles and less devotion to generalized theories like the Oedipus complex, if we were truly to reach those profoundly disturbed. Her determination to understand and to connect was truly legendary: it was said that she would have swung from the chandeliers if that would have helped her to help a patient.

Fromm-Reichmann embodied both of the focal points of this book: She devoted her entire working life to the care and cure of those considered hopeless by mainstream psychiatry and psychoanalysis, and she did this through a relentless pursuit of understanding that trusted the existence of a world common to both patient and therapist. Though she would never have used a word like *hermeneutics*—determined always to speak simply and directly, whether in English or in her native German—she lived a pragmatic hermeneutics that we can begin to characterize in this chapter. Both in her writings and from accounts of her clinical work (Chestnut Lodge records cited in Hornstein, 2000, and Greenberg, 1964), she maintained her conviction that schizophrenic speech and behavior do communicate, if only someone tries persistently enough to understand. This someone, however, had to remain constantly aware of countertransference, that is, of one's own history-shaped participation and contributions to the patient's experience. Thus, as Ferenczi had first insisted, the analysis of the analyst became indispensable. She believed it kept us clinicians aware of our common humanity, including those anxieties specifically triggered in our work with seriously disturbed people, so that we have a greater possibility of staying with them.

In this vein, Fromm-Reichmann's biographer Gail Hornstein (2000) wrote of the basic attitudes that, in my view, argue for her inclusion in the school of trust-hermeneutics:

> For Frieda, treatment of mental illness was like physical therapy after stroke: a painstaking exercise in hope. Improvement was unpredictable, and was often followed by relapse or deterioration. Recovery, to the extent it was present, proceeded at an agonizingly slow pace. It was natural for the doctor to have periods of discouragement, even real despair, but he couldn't afford to give up, no matter how many setbacks there were. *A patient had to have at least one person who could imagine the possibility of his getting well.* (pp. xvii–xviii, emphasis added)

In short, in Frieda Fromm-Reichmann we find a life given to the psychologically most destitute suffering strangers on the one hand and a life of embodied dialogic hermeneutics on the other.

LIFE AND WORK

Frieda Fromm-Reichmann, known to friends, colleagues, and patients simply as Frieda, was born in Karlsruhe, in the west of Germany in 1889.* The eldest of three daughters of a not-too-successful father and of the formidable Klara, in an Orthodox

---

* For the most part I have depended for biographical information on Hoffmann (1998) and on Hornstein (2000).

Jewish family, Frieda early understood how unobtrusively to keep the family functioning, a role she continued to play throughout life in institutions she did and did not manage. When she was nine, the family moved to Königsburg in eastern Prussia, where Klara's connections created better opportunities for the family. Both parents became deaf—her mother in Frieda's childhood—as Frieda did in her last years herself.

Though girls could not attend gymnasium, Klara saw to her daughters' education. Thus a well-prepared Frieda entered university and medical school at a time when this was extremely unusual for a girl. Less than 5 feet tall and a young woman in militaristic Prussia, she managed to excel and to impress as more than capable of every job for which she ever applied. Throughout her life she attributed her success to "hard work" and seems to have believed that anyone who worked as much could do as much. Nevertheless she always credited her teachers and mentors, among whom she counted Freud, Kurt Goldstein, Georg Groddeck, and Harry Stack Sullivan, and considered herself to play a secondary role: "I've had a life where I always had to be the muse, because I thought what they will do will be of greater significance. And what I could do was just to take off their jobs so that they could do their special work" (Silver & Fromm-Reichmann, 1989, p. 475). How much of this understated assessment of her own importance concerned gender roles during her lifetime would be hard to say; some of it clearly expressed an unassuming personal style. Asked how she had learned so much about people, she responded, "By observing my friends and relatives" (Szalita, 2001, p. 97).

Already during the First World War, working with brain-injured soldiers, she had developed the attitudes toward suffering human beings that shaped all her future work:

> When I was an intern at the psychiatric hospital of the medical school of the University of Königsberg, nobody knew yet what psychotherapy was. But I knew it could be done. What I did was to sit with the psychotics. Day and night, night and day, and listen to them and just say a few kind things so that they went on. I got

furious when they were mistreated. For instance, one day when we made rounds, first the big boss and then all the associates, there was a man who didn't take off his cap as the great professor came in. One of the attendants or the head nurse asked him, "Why don't you take off your cap?" And he said, "But I can't. These birds which I have there underneath my cap will fly." And everybody laughed to no end. I was so mad I could have killed them, because I knew it meant something. (Silver & Fromm-Reichmann, 1989, pp. 474–475)

When she went to hear "the great Kraepelin,"* she "was outraged about the way he did his talk in the presence of the patient about his epileptic seizures, about the epileptic character … what an invasion of the dignity of the man, the way he presented him!" (p. 474).

Later, working in Dresden (1920–1923) at the Weisser Hirsch sanitarium, she began psychoanalysis with Wilhelm Wittenberg and later completed psychoanalytic training in Berlin with Hans Sachs. She also first met Erich Fromm in Dresden.

Her years in Germany (1889–1933) included study and collaboration for many years with pioneering neuropsychologist Kurt Goldstein (1878–1965) from whom she learned the organic and holistic approach that became gestalt psychology and that influenced her continuously. From him she learned to see symptoms as answers to problems posed to the organism by the environment. Sickness came from a disturbance of the connections between the organism and its world, not from something inside the organism. Goldstein—who had studied neurology, psychoanalysis, and phenomenology—contributed importantly to the development of gestalt psychology, and he always cast himself in the role of one who had to learn from the patient.

A second friendship and collaboration with Georg Groddeck, a specialist in psychosomatic medicine, contributed to her lifelong conviction that all symptoms carry meaning. In the course of this friendship, she spent time with Ferenczi, whose ideas about

---

* Emil Kraepelin (1856–1926), founder of modern biological psychiatry.

recognizing early trauma, about trying whatever might reach the most disturbed, about admitting one's own mistakes, also became formative background. She would later mention Groddeck as one source of her understanding that lack of physical contact could contribute to the profound loneliness at the core of some psychoses (Fromm-Reichmann, 1990). She learned from Groddeck to attend to the individual patient, to tolerate complexity, to avoid professional language, and to speak simply (Petratos, 1990). (Speaking to psychoanalysts, her patient Joanne Greenberg noted wryly that Fromm-Reichmann "didn't add a single technical word to the two-ton load you have to carry"; Green, 1967, p. 74.) As respectful as she remained in her teaching and writing toward Freud and the Freudians—never wanting to become an exile like Karen Horney or Harry Stack Sullivan—she clearly drew inspiration from Groddeck and Ferenczi, who placed the care of the patient before loyalty to any dogma.*

In the mid-1920s she had moved to Heidelberg to establish a sanatorium or therapeutic community for Orthodox Jews of her own. Erich Fromm, younger, also an Orthodox Jew, was briefly her patient there[†] and later her husband, though they lived together only a few years and divorced after both had escaped to the United States. Erich, in 1935, helped to find Frieda work at Chestnut Lodge in Rockville, Maryland, where she spent her remaining years until her sudden death in 1957.

Her Judaism also inspired a sense of responsibility for her patients and for the healing of the world. She and Erich Fromm

---

* Not that she found it easy to go her own way. In the words of her friend Alberta Szalita (1981), "Frieda, because she relied on her empathic understanding, could come up with innovative interpretations; and these often disarmed her patients. But the psychoanalytic establishment took a negative attitude toward her efforts to adjust the classical psychoanalytic method to the therapeutic needs of schizophrenic patients. She was greatly hurt by this attitude and, because of the powerful influence of the psychoanalytic establishment, entertained fears of being identified as a heretic and cast out of the fraternity" (p. 13).

† In a late interview she said: "You see, I began to analyze Erich. And then we fell in love and so we stopped. That much sense we had! Erich and I married when I was 36, and we married in the middle of the sanatorium experience " (Silver & Fromm-Reichmann, 1989, p. 480).

had been part of the renewal of German Judaism, and their friends in Heidelberg seem to have included Franz Rosenzwieg, Martin Buber, and Gershom Scholem. (Buber remained a close enough friend that he visited her at Chestnut Lodge weeks before her death. He had come to Washington, DC, to lecture, but she felt she would not be able to hear him.) In later years she rarely spoke of these resources, but those who knew her well realized both her terrible Holocaust losses and her spiritual foundations.

At Chestnut Lodge, a unique psychoanalytic hospital for the treatment of schizophrenics without shock or lobotomy, Fromm-Reichmann collaborated with Dexter Bullard, its owner and manager, to create a therapeutic community where no patient was considered beyond hope. The hospital attempted to embody a deep respect for psychiatric patients, an unusual project then and now. Because everyone—even including nurses—was in analysis, sensitivity to meanings was intentionally extremely intense. No one escaped constant scrutiny. The emotional costs of working in such an atmosphere seem to have been large, but many patients—previously thought incurable—improved markedly, by their own later accounts.

In her later years, Fromm-Reichmann suffered from congenital deafness, became more and more depressed and withdrawn, and died at Chestnut Lodge in 1957 of acute coronary thrombosis. Though some of her closest friends suspected suicide, no clear evidence has ever been found for this conclusion. In her autobiographical tape recording, Fromm-Reichmann said clearly that she believed her father's death at the bottom of an elevator shaft in 1926 was his own doing: "I still think he did it. He was very deaf" (Silver, 1996, p. 41).

After her death, Joanne Greenberg published a fictional account of her treatment at Chestnut Lodge with "Dr. Fried" titled *I Never Promised You a Rose Garden* as a testimony to the belief that the seriously mentally ill can improve to the point of living well in the world. Understated, unafraid of madness, Fromm-Reichmann remained continually available, trusting the patient and the process between them. When the patient asked, "You never were a mental patient, were you?" she responded,

> No ... I am sorry, too, because I can only guess at what it must be like. But it will not stop me from being able to help you. Only it makes it your responsibility to explain everything fully to me and to be a little patient with me if sometimes my perceptions are a bit slow ... I think now, though, that you are a little too happy with yourself for this trouble you have. I think you are giving up too easily, so let me say again that I will not betray you.

"Prove it!" shouted her patient. Fromm-Reichmann said, "A hard proof, but a valid one. Time" (Greenberg, 1964, p. 143).

Almost everyone who knew Fromm-Reichmann affirmed this book as a faithful portrait.

FROMM-REICHMANN'S HERMENEUTICS

No one description will adequately present Fromm-Reichmann's hermeneutics—her interpretive attitude—but a good place to start may be her hermeneutics of suffering. She often told the following story from her own clinical experience:

> I had worked with a patient for a long period of time. Despite her assaultiveness a good mutual working relationship had been established. One day, while she was in a wet pack, I asked her whether she would be willing to give a legally needed signature. Her prompt answer was, "if you unpack me." Turning away from the patient I walked toward the door of her room to go and ask the nurses to do so. On the verge of leaving the room I looked back at the patient without realizing why. I believed at the time, that as I looked back at her I caught the clue from the expression of disappointment and frustration, if not despair, on the patient's face, that "if you unpack me" meant me, and not the nurses. I came back and opened the pack singlehandedly, and she gave me her signature. Later on the patient related this experience as having been the first step toward her recovery. (Fromm-Reichmann, 1955a, p. 82)

Let us listen to Fromm-Reichmann's own interpretation of this incident, attending not so much to the patient's process as to her own. In retrospect, she believed that she had intuitively perceived the patient's desire before she had turned toward the door, but that "I had initially tried to suppress or repress the visual impression of the patient's misery as a source of my intuitive grasp of what she wanted" (p. 83). We can hear the Lévinasian struggle played out here, in exquisite honesty. She went on:

> I now believe I looked back because my sense of obligation toward the patient became stronger than the anxiety-born suppressive or repressive forces which previously were at work. I felt I had to overcome or ignore my anxiety and to react adequately to the message emanating from the patient's despair, which previously I had intuitively grasped in my initial observation of her unhappy facial expression. (p. 83)

Another basic hermeneutic principle was one that Fromm-Reichmann shared with Harry Stack Sullivan, that is, that we are all more simply human than otherwise. In practice, this meant two things to both of them, first, that the so-called mentally ill are people like us and understandable in the same terms:

> The first prerequisite for successful psychotherapy is the respect that the psychiatrist must extend to the mental patient. Such respect can be valid only if the psychiatrist realizes that his patient's difficulties in living are not too different from his own. (Fromm-Reichmann, 1950, p. xi)
>
> The fact that a person needs psychiatric help in handling his emotional difficulties in living by no means constitutes any basic inferiority. Only the psychiatrist who realizes this is able to listen to his patients in such a way that there may be psychotherapeutic success. (p. 17)

Second, it meant that we are all best understood as struggling to cope with terrible anxieties and that everything we do and say, and whatever we do that seems extremely strange, begins to make sense in these terms. This, I think, was Fromm-Reichmann's form of the hermeneutic circle, the reading of the whole from the parts and the parts from the whole. She read our common humanity from its particular anxieties in individual human sufferers, including herself, and from the idiosyncratic and individual she formed and maintained her sense of common humanity.

Finally, we must acknowledge that Fromm-Reichmann's hermeneutics, unlike those of the interpersonal school (here-and-now emphasis) with which she is usually identified, were profoundly developmental and in quite a different direction from the predominant Freudian and Kleinian psychoanalysis of her time. She seems not to have been well acquainted with the independent voices in British psychoanalysis like Fairbairn, Winnicott, and Bowlby who have become so influential for clinical developmentalists today.* But she had read widely in her search for understanding of terrible anxieties, and she mentioned Klein, Sharpe, Spitz, Ferenczi, Rank, Freud, Rado, Sullivan, Fromm, Horney, and Silverberg (in that order; Fromm-Reichmann, 1954, p. 718) as among those she had read in her search, without saying what she thought of which sources. She concluded, "*The feeling of powerlessness, of helplessness in the presence of inner dangers, which the individual cannot control*, constitutes in the last analysis the common background of all further elaborations on the theory of anxiety" (p. 718, emphasis added). She went on to explicate her own hypothesis on the developmental origins of anxiety. I quote it at length because it illustrates not only the content of her thinking but her straightforward, jargon-free, no-nonsense way of understanding people (hermeneutics) and way of talking:

> The most universal source of inner helplessness in adults, I believe, stems from their unresolved fixations to the emotional entanglements with significant persons of their early lives, in our culture, of course, mainly with parents during childhood. The result of

---

* Her posthumously published "Loneliness" (1990), however, contains extensive references to Suttie (1988), indicating another source of her developmental sensibility: "As Suttie has put it, separation from the direct tenderness and nurtural love relationship with the mother may outrun the child's ability for making substitutions. This is a rather serious threat to an infant and child in a world where a taboo exists on tenderness among adults. When such a premature weaning from mothering tenderness occurs the roots for permanent aloneness and isolation, for 'love-shyness,' as Suttie has called it, for fear of intimacy and tenderness, are planted in the child's mind; and the defensive counterreactions against this eventuality may lead to psychopathological developments" (p. 311).

these fixations is that people compulsively appraise other people in terms of their ancient childhood patterns of living, judgments and expectations. They act upon and respond to people in line with these misconceptions. Many times people are half aware of their erroneous judgments, expectations and behavior, yet are helpless in their attempt to change. This is due to their lack of awareness of the unconscious roots of their compulsive need to repeat old patterns of relatedness and of living, i.e., of the unresolved fixations to their early ways of living with the significant people of their childhood. This helplessness in the face of the need for change of anachronistically distorted patterns meets with discontent and disapproval by oneself and others and—also frequently with hatred against anonymous and undefinable forces or, personified, against the people of the past who seem responsible for one's being held back against one's will. This powerlessness ... produces deep emotional insecurity in people. That is, it is the cause and the expression of anxiety. (Fromm-Reichmann, 1954, pp 718–719)

She was also curious about the differences reported between the civilian survivors of the London Blitzkrieg, few of whom became mental patients, and the survivors of family violence. She thought, with Ferenczi*—though she did not mention him in this connection—that the child was required to forget the origins of his or her profound anxieties, leaving trauma unspoken and unprocessed. In Hornstein's (2000) words, "Casualties in a war that was invisible, psychotics were thus in the terrifying position of trying to protect themselves from angers other people claimed weren't there" (p. 123).

---

* My collaborators would later speak of this origin of dynamic unconsciousness, one of the three forms they identified, besides prereflective and the unvalidated unconsciousness (Stolorow, Atwood, & Brandchaft, 1987): "The specific intersubjective contexts in which conflict takes form are those in which central affect states of the child cannot be integrated because they fail to evoke the requisite attuned responsiveness from the caregiving surround. Such unintegrated affect states become the source of lifelong inner conflict, because they are experienced as threats both to the person's established psychological organization and to the maintenance of vitally needed ties. Thus affect-dissociating defensive operations are called into play, which reappear in the analytic situation in the form of resistance. ... It is in the defensive walling off of central affect states, rooted in early derailments of affect integration, that the origins of what has traditionally been called the dynamic unconscious can be found" (pp. 91–92).

Perhaps the best way to get a sense of Frieda Fromm-Reichmann's hermeneutics of trust in the humanity of the seriously disturbed patient, that is, in the world we share (Dostal, 1987), is to listen to her explaining the schizophrenic's struggle:

> During the early fight for emotional survival, the schizophrenic begins to develop the great interpersonal sensitivity that remains for the rest of his or her life. Initial psychogenic experiences are actually, or by virtue of interpretation, the pattern for a never-ending succession of subsequent similar ones. Finally, the schizophrenic transgresses the threshold of endurance. Because of the sensitivity and the never-satisfied, lonely need for benevolent contact, this threshold is all too easily reached.
>
> The schizophrenic's special emotional regression and withdrawal from the outside world into an autistic private world with its specific thought processes and modes of feeling and expression are motivated by a fear of repetitional rejection, distrust of others, and a fear of losing the boundaries between the self and others. ... That is, schizophrenics fear losing their shaky personal identities. In addition, they are equally afraid of their own hostilities, which they abhor, as well as of the deep anxieties promoted by their hatred. (Fromm-Reichmann & Silver, 1990, p. 54)

Fromm-Reichmann understood the mental patient not as an alien but as a fellow human being with experiences that concern regular human suffering: desperate need for benevolent contact, sensitivity, fear of their own hostility, anxiety. We hear the resonant voice of the hermeneutics of generous compassion and trust, so difficult to maintain in the face of the pressures of a psychiatric hospital.

So we can say the following about Fromm-Reichmann's hermeneutics in general: (a) She attended always to her personal clinical experience, including what is commonly called countertransference; (b) though she always gave Freud credit for inventing psychoanalysis and directing us to unconscious processes, her theoretical understanding was strongly Sullivanian with its alternate view of development, its replacement of instincts and drives with interpersonal processes, and its more restricted understanding of the sexual; (c) her reading, however, as noted previously, was wide and inclusive and kept her hermeneutic circle an expanding one; and (d) in the end, her voice, while never that of a closed view, was always identifiably her own, clear, direct, and unapologetic. She saw the disturbed people who smeared feces as her humiliated neighbors. Supervisees like Anna Gourevitch have described her attitudes:

> She unquestionably taught me not to disregard anything which seemed to me as irrelevant. She took into account every detail. It was impressive—the respect she had for the patient's communications of any kind. She was never judgmental. She tried to understand. It didn't make any difference whether she liked or didn't like the patient. She treated them all with the same seriousness and concern. (Szalita, 2001, p. 96)

Alberta Szalita (2001) also reported that Fromm-Reichmann similarly accepted the therapist's angry feelings when hit in the face with a pillow by a patient. True to the ethos of Chestnut Lodge—largely shaped by Fromm-Reichmann—Szalita went on to remember in her own analysis being dominated in pillow fights with a brother. Everyone worked at understanding his or her own responses ("countertransferences") constantly so as to be able to meet the psychotic patients in their care.

CLINICAL SENSIBILITY

Fromm-Reichmann followed only two guidelines in her practice: (a) find whatever will work with this particular patient, and (b) trust as your guide the patient's own capacity for healing. In her own description,

> Even when these people are completely in the throes of a severe disorder, they may at times still be quite capable of staying related to another person.
>
> I remember in this connection a patient who was sitting naked on the floor as I came in his room to see him. He was hallucinating, delusional, and seemingly out of touch, but as I came in, he pulled a blanket down from the bed and said, "I still know how to behave in the presence of a lady." His next sentence was, "Can you tell me, however, what made me go into this animal-like state?"

There followed a three-hour conversation during which I had trouble understanding the patient because he was talking very low, he had not eaten for several days, and his mouth was exceedingly dried out. So, I sat down on the floor with him in order to facilitate personal contact.

After three hours, I felt that I could ask him whether he would like to drink a little milk, because this seemed to be one of the emergent needs he had. I went and got some milk, and he took a sip. Then he threw the glass into my face, got terribly frightened, and again related to me, saying, "I told you it would be dangerous to come too close to me. See what I had to do. You had better leave the room, I don't know whether I may have to do more on that order." (Fromm-Reichmann & Silver, 1990, p. 53)

Fromm-Reichmann noticed and trusted this person's capacity to relate to her, as well as his concern for her. It was thus easier not to be offended and to come back the next day and to sit with him, to ask him, a "fellow sufferer," if it would be safe to sit with him today, and so on. She insisted that "the less fear patients sense in the therapist, the less dangerous they are" (Hornstein, 2000, p. 48). For 22 years at Chestnut Lodge, she patiently accompanied and worked psychoanalytically (no shock treatments) with her fellow human beings and helped her colleagues to understand what prevented them from doing as she did.

Similarly, she understood that any symptom, if the therapist received it in a matter-of-fact spirit, could be workable because it would turn out to carry meaning:

A schizophrenic young woman was given to compulsive anal masturbation, followed by touching herself and her therapist with her hands, which were soiled with fecal matter. The psychoanalyst could not help resent having her arms and her dresses soiled by the patient. She dreaded therapeutic interviews with the girl until she decided to wear worn-out, long-sleeved washable dresses while seeing this patient.* There followed a marked feeling of relaxation on the part of the psychoanalyst, to which the schizophrenic girl

---

* This story reminds me of Sandra Buechler's (2009) words: "...We often have a particularly profound impact when our behavior says, 'I care more about helping you than I care about how I look '" (p. 65), though she surely refers to more than just physical appearance.

responded immediately by ceasing to smear feces. Soon she was able to participate in therapeutic discussions of her compulsory anal masturbation and to discontinue it. She has since recovered from her severe mental disorder. (Fromm-Reichmann, 1959, p. 141)

What happened here? The therapist—most likely Fromm-Reichmann herself—found a way to regard what the patient was doing as "no big deal" or at least as no offense to her. The focus shifted then to the patient's meanings, in a shift of gestalt, and a different dialogue could ensue. Fromm-Reichmann understood that the framework or prejudices that she brought to the dialogue were keeping it stuck, and she managed to dislodge them within a hermeneutic of trust in the communicative possibility of even such a symptom.

But the question remains: Not only how did she understand but what did she understand that made such persistent work possible? Let us turn for a clue to her posthumously published article on loneliness.

THE HERMENEUTICS OF INCOMMUNICABLE LONELINESS

It may seem odd to speak of a hermeneutics of loneliness, but I refer to a specific capacity for understanding and interpreting that Frieda Fromm-Reichmann brought to her work. She recognized a fundamental and lonely despair, as Winnicott would similarly recognize the fear of breakdown as the memory of a catastrophe long already occurred. She could see and hear it when it seemed to have no voice, and she gave it voice:

> Perhaps my interest began with the young catatonic woman who broke through a period of completely blocked communication and obvious anxiety by responding when I asked her a question about her feeling miserable: She raised her hand with her thumb lifted, the other four fingers bent toward her palm, so that I could see only the thumb, isolated from the four hidden fingers. I interpreted the signal with, "That lonely?" in a sympathetic tone of voice. At this, her facial expression loosened up as though in great relief and gratitude, and her fingers opened.

Then she began to tell me about herself by means of her fingers, and she asked me by gestures to respond in kind. We continued with this finger conversation for one or two weeks, and as we did so, her anxious tension began to decrease and she began to break through her noncommunicative isolation; and subsequently she emerged altogether from her loneliness. (Fromm-Reichmann, 1990, p. 305)

Fromm-Reichmann explained that the overwhelming loneliness she recognized[*] in schizophrenics differed profoundly from transient or productive aloneness or even existential aloneness before an important choice or in the face of our human finitude. It resembles more an unreachable and unspeakable despair:

The more severe developments of loneliness appear in the unconstructive, desolate phases of isolation and real loneliness which are beyond the state of feeling sorry for oneself—the states of mind in which the fact that there were people in one's past life is more or less forgotten, and the possibility that there may be interpersonal relationships in one's future life is out of the realm of expectation or imagination. This loneliness, in its quintessential form, is of such a nature that it is incommunicable by one who suffers it. Unlike other noncommunicable emotional experiences, it cannot even be shared empathically, perhaps because the other person's empathic abilities are obstructed by the anxiety-arousing quality of the mere emanations of this profound loneliness. (Fromm-Reichmann, 1990, p. 312)

This last sentence calls for special attention. My own anxiety before the face of the other this destitute, as Lévinas might have said, most often interferes with my responding in a way that makes a difference to the person so unspeakably alone. What this anxiety concerns, she does not really say—Lévinasian persecution, vicarious trauma, contagion?—but we do know she was less

---

[*] Ann-Louise Silver (1996, 1999) believes her capacity to pick up this kind of loneliness was connected to her familial and impending deafness and perhaps also to her deep and frustrated longing for children. For me these explanations could be only elements of a greater complexity.

afraid than most to name the loneliness when she recognized it. Probably she was well acquainted with it herself.

> People who are in the grip of severe degrees of loneliness cannot talk about it; and people who have at some time in the past had such an experience can seldom do so either, for it is so frightening and uncanny in character that they try to dissociate the memory of what it was like, and even the fear of it. This frightened secretiveness and lack of communication about loneliness seems to increase its threat for the lonely ones, even in retrospect; it produces the sad conviction that nobody else has experienced or ever will sense what they are experiencing or have experienced. (Fromm-Reichmann, 1990, pp. 313–314)

Sometimes responding to this naked destitution of the vulnerable face precisely means acknowledging that no words can express the depth of the loneliness or the terror—that it is incommunicable. She went on:

> Even mild borderline states of loneliness do not seem to be easy to talk about. Most people who are alone try to keep the mere fact of their aloneness a secret from others, and even try to keep its conscious realization hidden from themselves. I think that this may be in part determined by the fact that loneliness is a most unpopular phenomenon in this group-conscious culture. Perhaps only children have the independence and courage to identify their own loneliness as such—or perhaps they do it simply out of a lack of imagination or an inability to conceal it. One youngster asked another, in the comic strip *Peanuts*, "Do you know what you're going to be when you grow up?" "Lonesome," was the unequivocal reply of the other. (Fromm-Reichmann, 1990, p. 314)

It seems to me that she suggests here that the incommunicable loneliness results from a missing developmental experience resembling what Winnicott (1958a) described in "The Capacity to Be Alone." In the context of the mother's sustaining but nonintrusive presence, the child learns that aloneness can be a space of creative aliveness. Absent this experience, aloneness accumulates as terror and despair. Some find themselves in worlds of delusion where they despair of ever finding understanding; others sink, as perhaps did Fromm-Reichmann herself, into depressive isolation where darkness seems to close in around them.

Her critics, and previous tradition, had claimed that psychotic patients' tendency to act instead of speak meant they could not form transferences—those intense relational relivings seen as central to psychoanalytic process since the time of Freud and Dora. Therefore these patients remained beyond the reach of psychoanalytic clinicians, at that time left to crude versions of shock therapy, lobotomies, and back wards of state hospitals. Frieda Fromm-Reichmann's hermeneutic of trust saw in their lonely faces the capacity to love and be loved, and this sustained her hope.

> One of our patients at Chestnut Lodge, as she emerged from a severe state of schizophrenic depression, asked to see me because she wished to tell me about the deep state of hopeless loneliness and subjective isolation which she had undergone during her psychotic episodes. But even though she was now in fine command of the language, and even though she came with the intention of talking, she was just as little able to tell me about her loneliness in so many words as are most people who are engulfed in or have gone through a period of real psychotic loneliness. After several futile attempts, she finally burst out, "I don't know why people think of hell as a place where there is heat and where fires are burning. That is not hell. Hell is if you are frozen in isolation into a block of ice. That is where I have been." (Fromm-Reichmann, 1990, p. 319)

We will find that Winnicott and others—surely some of my patients—describe traumatic and posttraumatic states as freezing. Perhaps this profound and incommunicable loneliness concerns a despair that any exit from this freezing, or even any understanding of it, will be possible. After all, understanding would warm it a little bit. Fromm-Reichmann continued,

> I don't know whether this patient was familiar with Dante's description of the ninth and last, or frozen circle of the Inferno. It is in essence quite similar to the patient's conception of hell—the "lowest part of the Universe, and farthest remote from the Source of all light and heat," reserved for the gravest sinners, namely

those "who have done violence to their own kindred (like Cain who slew Abel), and those who committed treachery against their native land." Among others, Dante met there "two sinners that are frozen close together in the same hole." (pp. 319–320)

Unfortunately we clinicians, as Fromm-Reichmann knew well, often fear being frozen together with our patients in the same lonely hole. This anxiety keeps us from touching theirs, for even if we find our courage and join them, we may stay too close. Fromm-Reichmann's colleague Alberta Szalita (2001) cautioned, "It is good to be able to put yourself into someone else's shoes, but you have to remember that you don't wear them" (p. 100).

As protection from the anxiety that keeps us from approaching our patient's frozen loneliness, I particularly recommend meditation on the last section of Sandra Buechler's "The Analyst's Experience of Loneliness" (1998), in which she extensively considers Fromm-Reichmann's essay. She titled this section "The Analyst's Capacity to Be Alone." Here is an excerpt, clearly addressing both Fromm-Reichmann and those of us who want to work in her spirit:

> How can we analysts, long-distance runners that we all must be, avoid at least some of this loneliness? Of course, our own character types and early experiences play a significant role in our vulnerability to loneliness when alone. How able we are to retain a sense of self in the absence of confirmation or in the presence of disconfirmation depends on *both* of our developmental histories: our early, childhood separation-individuation and identity formation experiences, and our later, analytic separation-individuation and identity formation experiences. These histories are, I suggest, equally important. (pp. 110–111)

Our own history most often comes into psychoanalytic discussion under the rubric of countertransference—both troublesome and inevitable but also potentially creative. Buechler suggested, in addition, that our double history (personal and analytic) provides the resources, the repertoires, the set of internal voices we need to support us every day as clinicians:

> The internal chorus we bring into our offices every day must be of comfort, and must be sufficiently stimulating, to encourage the creative use of aloneness. The feeling the chorus must give us is that whatever may go on today, with this particular patient, does not define us as analysts, for we have already been defined and have defined ourselves, through our analytic identifications and identity formation. We are not personally and professionally at stake with each new interaction with a patient. With this foundation, we can experience aloneness with a patient as information, rather than as judgment. We can turn the aloneness over in our minds, wonder what it is about, become curious about it, see it as meaningful, as something to understand, but not as an obstacle or an indictment. An aloneness that doesn't cost us a good connection with ourselves, with our chorus, or with the patient can be used creatively. A creatively used aloneness is not loneliness. (p. 111)

In other words, Buechler suggested, embracing and using our experiences of aloneness in clinical work can support our work, not leave us and the patient in our frozen hell. She clearly knows that this is not the same loneliness of which Fromm-Reichmann wrote but rather a more Winnicottian aloneness in the presence of our psychoanalytic vocation, of our virtual community. Buechler holds out hope that creative use of aloneness can perhaps reach those who live in the incommunicable despair:

> To be alone while with a patient is not painful, so long as we can retain a connection with a good sense of self, and a nonpersecutory sense of the patient. Theoretical concepts can aid this process, by providing something to play with during alone times with the patient. A good, supportive internal chorus and enough to play with can, I believe, allow the analyst creative possibilities for the productive use of aloneness. (p. 110)

Whether Fromm-Reichmann would have agreed is hard to say; she spoke more often of intuition and hard work.

It seems to me that a strong sense of one's connections to others beyond one's work is also crucial. In Fromm-Reichmann's last years, her two sisters lived in Israel, many of her closest friends had died, and deafness cut her off from human conversation. She seems to have made more creative use of her own loneliness to touch others when she could still participate in conversation. She seems to have written this posthumously published article when darkness was overtaking her.

We may reasonably ask whether devotion to our work, to relief of human suffering at the level we see in the life of Frieda Fromm-Reichmann, Sándor Ferenczi, and Donald Winnicott, leads inevitably to burnout and despair. No easy question is this. As far as I can tell, each of them responded to what seemed completely imperative and had no regrets about the costs to themselves. (It is hard to say what their sacrifice cost their significant others, though Gizella Ferenczi and Clare Winnicott seem to have understood very well what their partners were doing and to have accompanied them firmly if not always enthusiastically.) Buechler suggests that we can work in their spirit and yet use our own personal and communal resources to support us better. Surely not all of us actually can be such pathbreakers, but our remembrance of their courage can become part of the "internal chorus" that sustains us in our own darker and lonelier periods.

FLEXIBLE THERAPEUTIC BOUNDARIES AND TRUST

Of the five therapists this book considers, only Fromm-Reichmann tackled in print the question of rules and boundaries. Each of our five pioneers was known to have behaved in unorthodox ways for the sake of helping patients; she was unafraid to say so, to say why, and to explain when to be concerned. Let us listen and comment [in brackets]:

> It used to be considered most important that patients in analysis have not even an accidental meeting with the analyst outside his office; consequently, the patients reacted to any such accidental meeting with intensive emotional reactions. [*Note that as in the smearing instance above, the therapist's attitude often makes something a problem or not.*] This does not mean the advocacy of relinquishing the principle of a strictly professional relationship

132 • The Suffering Stranger

between doctor and patient or a denial of the wisdom of avoiding extra-professional meetings with certain patients [*not all*] who are, at times, so overwhelmed by their current problems that they should be protected from any possibility of additional emotional complexities. [*Here there is a strong sense of "it depends," conceding that in many instances complexities will be either unavoidable or even the lesser of evils.*] The quality and number of these difficulties are largely dependent upon whether the psychoanalyst expects them to occur and whether he creates the expectation of their occurrence in the patient. [*Once again, if meeting my patient at a professional meeting is something that I treat as a normal event, it is unlikely to become traumatic for the patient, though I may inquire about meanings.*] The psychoanalyst is justified in safeguarding his private life and his leisure against professional interference, provided—if the issue arises—that he gives the patient no false rationalizations as reasons. [*Like Ferenczi, she knew that patients hear our hypocrisy.*] However, the psychoanalyst who feels so keenly about his personal needs that he cannot endure making occasional exceptions is not suited for psychotherapy with hospitalized psychotics. There is no place in psychoanalysis—be it in ambulatory or hospital practice—for a state of splendid isolation to maintain the patient's transference-glorification of his therapist to bolster the latter's security. [*This is no profession for those who want an easy life, protected from the needs of the suffering other, or for anyone who wants to be important.*] (1959, p. 142)

This paragraph sounds simple, but its complexity astounds. She trusted the wise and generous therapist, in a collaborative spirit, to find the right boundaries with a particular patient, to protect but not overprotect the therapist's own life, to live humbly and generously. This combination meant noting the old rules (the "thou shalt nots"),* like cautionary signposts, but keeping one's eyes and ears open to respond as creatively as

---

* For readers who did not grow up in the psychoanalytic tradition, these rules included the following: The patient must lie on the couch. The analyst must sit behind the patient, out of view. The patient must say everything that comes to mind. The analyst must interpret, but remain neutral and anonymous. The analyst must maintain the "frame" (i.e., the exact time, agreed-upon fee). There will be no contact outside the analytic hours. The analyst does not answer questions, but interprets them. The analyst does not accept gifts, but interprets them. There is no physical contact, except in Europe, where a handshake at the beginning and end of session is normal.

possible to the patient. "Every patient came to treatment with unique needs; to reduce him to a disease entity was an insult to his humanity and a sign of the doctor's lack of imagination" (Hornstein, 2000, p. 43). Fromm-Reichmann herself was known to take patients to the symphony in Washington, DC, among other unorthodox proceedings. Her first question to a patient was "How can I help you?" This is not the question of someone who already knows in advance how to work according to the rules. Her hermeneutics of trust meant trusting both her own intuitive process (Fromm-Reichmann, 1955b) and the patient's natural resiliency and desire to recover, even when neither was immediately evident. The therapist's task was to maintain and offer hope.

Biographer Gail Hornstein interviewed Joanne Greenberg, Fromm-Reichmann's patient and author of *I Never Promised You a Rose Garden*. Greenberg spoke of Fromm-Reichmann's playfulness, her willingness to admit mistakes, her trust in her patient, and, above all, her capacity to create a sense of safety for one whose world had never been safe: "The trouble with mental illness is that it's drowning. You can't see above the water. You can't see what's past the pain. You have no height. What the patient needs is for you to be able to see over there, to see that there's a shoreline" (Hornstein, 2000, p. 381).

Earlier, still speaking under her pseudonym "Hannah Green," Greenberg described facets of Fromm-Reichmann's working personality that capture her determination that people should be treated as people:

> She wasn't careful to hide her anger at the various idiocies of which the world is capable. I remember one incident in particular when, after one of the phone calls that peppered our sessions, she hung up and indulged in a string of remarks that was quite creditable, considering that English was a second language. She explained that she had been trying to convince the U.S. Immigration Service that insanity, when contracted at Buchenwald, should not be a bar to entry into the United States. After many letters and pleas on her part, the government

decided in favor of the letter of the law and the moral sanctity of its coastlines. Frieda had a cold seethe that was formidable, and because she shared bits of her joy and indignation, I was, even in the most brutal phases of illness, never an invalid. (Green, 1967, p. 75)

Clearly her willingness to be herself with her patients, a distinct deviation from traditional practice in psychoanalysis, allowed them to stay in contact with their own humanity when others had exiled them. No matter how ill, Greenberg remained for Fromm-Reichmann a human being with whom she could expostulate about the idiocies of the American government. In Greenberg's experience—and this was no contradiction for either of them—Fromm-Reichmann put nothing before the care of the patient:

> In spite of her talk about psychotherapy being a science, she had little of the professionalistic cant that puts *any* theory ahead of a patient. I believe she would swing from the chandelier like Tarzan if she thought it would help; and she knew the book well enough to throw it away, or at least not to read it while the patient was watching. It must be difficult not to exploit patients to prove a theory—I know it happens in your profession and in others—but Frieda never did it to me and I am grateful. (p. 76)

Greenberg's remark about never reading the book while the patient was watching reminds me of Gadamer's "disappearing interpretation."* Fromm-Reichmann had been reading and thinking psychoanalysis for her entire adult life by the time she met Joanne Greenberg and her other Chestnut Lodge patients. She had also been trying to understand the human experiences of brain-injured soldiers and patients rejected and abandoned by

---

* In Chapter 1, we discussed Gadamer's conception of the "disappearing interpretation": "Paradoxically, an interpretation is right when it is capable of disappearing in this way. And yet at the same time it must be expressed as something that is supposed to disappear" (Gadamer, Weinsheimer, & Marshall, 2004, p. 399). The interpretation disappears both because the concepts used to make it have become part of the shared world and because the interlocutors have participated in the process of understanding to the extent that neither appears as the interpreter.

traditional psychoanalysis for all of those years. She had come to realize that only through the most rigorous honesty with herself and sincerity with her patients was it possible to reach the suffering other. Then the concepts behind the interpretive work tended to disappear and make it all look deceptively simple. She believed that anyone—honest and hardworking enough—could work as she did, without realizing that the unique combination of intuitive capacity developed in her family, keen intelligence, and moral and spiritual commitment to the most vulnerable set a very high standard. She did, however, know the costs: that the clinician too must bear the incommunicable loneliness. We are in her debt.

THE COSTS OF VOCATIONAL COMMITMENT

Lives like those of Ferenczi and Fromm-Reichmann remind me of book titles like Dietrich Bonhoeffer's *The Cost of Discipleship* (1995) and Chris Jaenicke's *The Risks of Relatedness* (2008). Orchestra conductors and philosophers do generally seem to live longer than these clinicians we are considering here, of whom only Brandchaft has lived beyond the age of 78, and both Ferenczi and Fromm-Reichmann died much younger. Working on this book has forced me to consider where longevity ranks among my values. It seems to me that we owe it to our patients, our significant others, and ourselves to care and provide for our physical and mental health as well as we can and better in some ways than did these groundbreakers. On the other hand, all of them were culturally rich people who enjoyed music, literature, and friendship, as well as wine and, unfortunately in some cases, tobacco. I do not believe there is any way, if we extend ourselves beyond what has been considered "appropriate" for our suffering patients, to guarantee that we will not suffer with them and that we may not die younger as a result. Frieda Fromm-Reichmann clearly did not feel sorry for herself: "So, if you want to know something for my epitaph, then I think we could say I wasn't lazy and I had lots of fun, but of another type as compared with many other people. It was a special type of fun" (Silver & Fromm-Reichmann, 1989, p. 481).

5

D. W. Winnicott
Humanitarian Without Sentimentality

We are poor indeed if we are only sane.

—**Winnicott**

...success in infant care depends on the fact of devotion, not on cleverness or intellectual enlightenment.

—**Winnicott**

Donald Woods Winnicott,* both insider and outsider, but ultimately giant of British psychoanalysis, remains an enigmatic figure. His original contributions to psychoanalysis and to the understanding of children have made him perhaps the psychoanalyst most quoted around the world, often Freud included. His lifelong determination to speak in his own voice makes him hard to classify, except as a true "independent." His transgressions keep him hard to admire without ambivalence. Here, however, we will consider him as a psychoanalytic hermeneut, a very visual interpreter who taught us to see and hear differently. Above all, he taught us to see clinically through the eyes of very young children, to notice the longings and distress of children in the faces of our

---

* The felicitous description, "humanitarian without sentimentality," comes from historian of psychoanalysis Paul Roazen (1997).

adult patients, and to see and feel their missing caregivers, full of love and hate, in ourselves.

The work of Winnicott illustrates both the importance and the hazards of everything that this book concerns. His playful trust in the squiggle* game to bring out important emotional truth from dialogic engagement provides the best nonverbal example possible of Gadamerian hermeneutics and of what this entire book means by a hermeneutics of trust. Furthermore, to see photographs of him working with children, or to read Margaret Little's account of her analysis with him, is to glimpse what Lévinasian responding to the face of the other could actually mean in clinical work. We can see how he extended himself and gave meaning to words like *substitution* and *transcendence*. Something—I leave this deliberately vague—looks luminous when we regard *his* face. Historian of psychoanalysis Paul Roazen described him as by far the most open and gracious of all the psychoanalysts he ever interviewed.

But we know there was a dark side, and in the case of Winnicott, we cannot evade it. The biographical aspects I will leave to the biographers, for the most part. The unavoidable question is whether the dangers of hubristic overreaching inhere in the humanistic therapeutics we consider in this book and thus whether the rules and protections Freud instituted remain wise, after all. Or is it possible to learn from our humanists and maintain the needed fallibilistic humility that can protect us from the "ruthlessness" that can become recklessness? I leave these questions open as we begin.

LIFE AND WORK

Born in 1896 to a prosperous Methodist but generally playful and nonconformist family,† Donald Woods Winnicott was the

---

* "In this squiggle game I make some kind of an impulsive line-drawing and invite the child whom I am interviewing to turn it into something, and then he makes a squiggle for me to turn into something in my turn" (1971, p. 16).
† For biographical information I have depended on Kahr (1996), Neve (1992), Roazen (1997), and Rodman (2003).

youngest of three, with two older sisters. With his locally prominent merchant father, his more capable parent though too much absent, he shared his religious spirit but no interest in commerce. His father realized that Donald needed to be sent away to school, where he thrived. At home, where he often returned, he felt—as he later wrote—that he was always keeping his depressed mother alive.

Always full of life—Roazen (1997) described him as a man of "buoyantly spontaneous charm"—he engaged in sports, read voraciously, especially Darwin and Freud, and played piano, especially Bach, all his life. He studied medicine, specialized in pediatrics, and became a pediatric psychiatrist. One of the first candidates in the Institute of Psychoanalysis in London, he began his training analysis with James Strachey, and later, because Melanie Klein refused to accept him for a second analysis (she wanted him to analyze her son), he did a second analysis with Joan Riviere. Neither, he felt, reached the trouble with his mother.

After medical school, he had married the fragile Alice Taylor, with whom he remained until after his father died in 1949. By then he had had two psychoanalyses, two heart attacks, and a long affair with Clare Britton, who became his second wife, and he had begun to contribute important papers to psychoanalysis. His many years working in pediatrics had given him a unique standpoint on the psychoanalytic situation, and in the 1950s this perspective increasingly isolated him from the dominant Kleinians in the British Psychoanalytic Society. After Klein's death in 1960, Anna Freud came to see him as having views closer to her own, but he remained independent until his own death in 1971. Because he belonged to neither camp, he was rarely allowed to teach candidates in the British Society, though he regularly delivered and discussed papers there. In the last 10 years of his life, he was well-known internationally and, despite ill health, continued to work intensively with very disturbed patients and to write important and creative papers. Historian of psychoanalysis Paul Roazen (1997) wrote,

> Even though concepts of Winnicott's, such as that of the "transitional object," became widely accepted, in 1968 he was so roughly received at the New York Psychoanalytic Society that he returned to his hotel room where he had a serious coronary attack that he spent months recovering from. (He had already experienced heart seizures, but the reception he got in New York was a shock.) Winnicott saw the relationship between analyst and patient in terms which were too interpersonal for orthodox American analytic thinking then. (In the mid-1960s Winnicott told me in an interview that he thought it was impossible to get properly analyzed in the States.) Winnicott was willing to tolerate almost psychotic-sounding regressions in analysands for the pursuit of a "true self," yet he remained unusually constructive in outlook and exceptionally generous in supportiveness. (pp. 207–208)

The sheer volume of his work is second only to that of Freud. He died in 1971.*

The famous and infamous Masud Kahn, who arrived in London from Pakistan in 1945, Winnicott's analysand for an indeterminate number of years, also edited most of Winnicott's work that appeared in his lifetime. This brilliant man seems to have deteriorated during and after his work with Winnicott (Kahr, 2003), committed numerous egregious ethical violations, and was ultimately expelled from the British Society. As biographer Brett Kahr (2003) noted, many considerations ought perhaps to have prevented Winnicott from taking Kahn as a patient, especially including the preexisting complexity of their relationship (though such situations were common in early psychoanalysis and sometimes unavoidable today). But using a patient—even a former patient—as editor seems not to have bothered Winnicott. In hindsight, we can say that he should have worried, as perhaps Freud, practitioner of the school of suspicion, should have worried about his own motives in using his patient Strachey (Winnicott's first analyst, by the way) as his translator and in analyzing his own daughter. What is it that misleads us into exploiting the therapeutic relationship,

---

* Death, he thought, had nothing to do with a "death instinct"; instead, "death is a disaster, which you have to put up with, because you're human" (Neve, 1992, p. 176).

even without sexual violations? The examples of both Freud and Winnicott force this question upon us, but let us suspend it for the moment.

WINNICOTT AS HERMENEUT

Our first hermeneutic task in reading Winnicott is to guess at the meaning of words he used in ways that seem seductively clear but are not at all.* His determination to think everything out for himself kept him from reading others much or from using language in easily recognizable ways. This was true of other first-generation analysts, and later original thinkers, but Winnicott was also thoughtful about language in ways that both can easily escape our notice and make us more aware. Consider this remark from his paper on countertransference:

> I think that the use of this word counter-transference should now be brought back to its original use. We can use words as we like, especially artificial words like counter-transference. A word like "self" naturally knows more than we do; it uses us, and can command us. But counter-transference is a term that we can enslave. (1965, p. 158)

In other words, instead of distinguishing between experience-near and experience-distant theorizing, as Heinz Kohut would do around the same time, Winnicott distinguished between everyday language in which we live and which uses and commands us and the technical language we make up to serve our theoretical purposes. For him, an important hermeneutical attitude involved attention to this distinction, and a clear personal preference kept him in the murky world of everyday spoken language for the most part. When he returned to the world of psychoanalytic shoptalk, in order to communicate to that world, his writing often took on

---

* Thomas Ogden (2001) has contributed an amazing study of the interaction between content and style in Winnicott's writing, specifically attending to his "Primitive Emotional Development" (1945); see also Hopkins (1997).

the feel of one speaking a second language, from which he quickly returned to his own.

He remained more than willing to discard, with alacrity, the technical ideas and terms themselves when he found them unworkable: "The whole concept of narcissism leaves out the tremendous differences that result from the general attitude and behavior of the mother" (Winnicott, Winnicott, Shepherd, & Davis, 1989, p. 191).

Winnicott rarely compared his ideas with those of others, so that contextualizing them remains more than difficult. Thus, I would suggest, we approach him best via the famous hermeneutic circle, reading back and forth between whole and part. Each piece of his writing, and there are hundreds, can be taken as a shining gem, but this approach leaves us with hundreds of Winnicotts. On the other hand, reading him as a whole seems impossible, because despite his love for the music of Bach—he played it on the piano from memory—the assemblage of his favorite words seems to form not counterpoint but cacophony. Love and hate, generosity and destruction, maternal preoccupation and use: This sounds like 20th-century music, not the music he loved to play. So what are we to make of this complex mass of writing?

If we are even to begin, we must, in a pragmatist spirit, hold every interpretation of him lightly. Each reading tests, as Winnicott himself said, the limits of our understanding of him. In the spirit of the hermeneutic circle, we read a paper, early or late, and try to see it in the context of the whole. We look at the whole and test it against the parts. In this way, bit by bit, we understand bit by bit. Just as Freud continually frustrates any attempt to reduce his work to a formula, because it was always a work in progress, so does Winnicott thwart us.

To take a strain of ideas that runs from hate through ruthlessness to use, it remains unclear to me how literally he meant these ideas to be taken but entirely clear that he considered them indispensable to understanding human development. Consider *hate*: At times it seems to signify the simple "ouch" of a mother bitten by a nursing infant, at others the male aspect of every personality

(Winnicott et al., 1989), at times the reactive capacity of the true self (Winnicott, 1965), at times simple assertiveness. *Ruthlessness*, a word that generally sounds like a deliberate indifference to ethics, meant at least the attitude of the preethical baby who simply takes what it needs: "Looking back one can say: I was ruthless then! The stage is one that is pre-ruth" (Winnicott, 1992, p. 265). Later one becomes concerned, in the stage of ruth, for the person who has to provide what one takes. But toward the end of his life—the period of the famous "Use of an Object" (Winnicott et al., 1989)—ruthlessness becomes a lifelong attitude that is willing to destroy to make the other—"object," he says—usable. How much this ruthlessness, and the question of use and being used, enters into the "dark side" problems remains for me an unresolved question.

The question about literal or metaphorical meaning belongs to what I will later be calling the hermeneutics of complexity, including his treatment of paradox and illusion. He refused to clarify preemptively whether what we "must" ruthlessly hate or destroy (Orange, 2008a), in order to be ourselves, is the actual other or an illusory "object." He requires us to hold the complexity of his theorizing just as caregivers and therapists must hold their own feelings of hate until children and patients are old enough ("in the transference") to bear knowing what we have suffered for them (Winnicott, 1949). On one side, it is both just and unjust to engage him in philosophical discussions about internal "objects" and external others and the mix-ups and confusions created by speaking in these dichotomous terms. On the other hand, his playful and elusive refusal to engage in such dialogues allows us to consider whether his work provides an entry point into a genuinely phenomenological hermeneutics for developmental studies, for psychoanalysis, and for all the humanistic psychotherapies.

Winnicott sometimes employed the word *significance* to point to *complex meaning to someone*. Although this word does not appear often in his work, it always carried a sense of weight, of centrally organizing import. It evokes a contextual world, and meaningful density that transcends the simplicity of the sentence, and carries an almost Heideggerian worldedness or Merleau-Pontean intricacy.

> The loss of the internal mother, who has acquired for the infant the *significance* of an inner source of love and protection and of life itself, greatly strengthens the threat of loss of the actual mother. Furthermore, the infant who throws away the spatula—and I think the same applies to the boy [in Freud's *fort-da* game] with the cotton-reel—not only gets rid of an external and internal mother who has stirred his aggression and is being expelled (and yet can be brought back): in my opinion he also externalizes an internal mother whose loss is feared, so as to demonstrate to himself that this internal mother, now represented through the toy on the floor, has not vanished from his inner world, has not been destroyed by the act of incorporation, is still friendly and willing to be played with. And by all this the child revises his relations with things and people both inside and outside himself. (Winnicott, 1941, p. 248, emphasis added)

Here the import, or *significance*, refers to what Kleinians call internal objects, and what he called the internal mother, someone whose loss or continuance organizes the infant's entire emotional life, and shows up clearly as he observed thousands of infants and mothers in the "set situation" with the spatula. Similarly, he wrote,

> Fear of breakdown is a feature of *significance* in some of our patients, but not in others. From this observation, if it be a correct one, the conclusion can be drawn that fear of breakdown is related to the individual's past experience, and to environmental vagaries. At the same time there must be expected a common denominator of the same fear, indicating the existence of universal phenomena; these indeed make it possible for everyone to know empathetically what it feels like when one of our patients shows this fear in a big way. (Winnicott, 1974, p. 103, emphasis added)

We will return to the fear of breakdown—something he had come to understand through his work with regression and dependency, much like Ferenczi's "child-analysis in the analysis of adults"; here let us note his insistence on complexity of significance, an important feature of a sensibility that trusts the patient and refuses reductionistic categories and answers.

The deceptive simplicity of Winnicott's writing, as Ogden (2001) so eloquently teaches us, should not mislead us. No naïve interpreter, his hermeneutic itself is complex and dense. Still, a clear and central feature, ever more emergent during his mature years, was his *developmental understanding of regression*, the topic of our next sections. His trust in regression as a developmental search for psychological recovery set him apart forever from the school of suspicion. Seeing all of psychological life developmentally and systemically, together with his temperamental optimism, led him to trust the emergence of humanity in those most destroyed by relational trauma.

A HERMENEUTICS OF DEVELOPMENT

Winnicott, as we have already seen, interpreted everything developmentally. Everything was what it was becoming. Brooke Hopkins (1997) noted, for example, the centrality of *capacity* in his writing: "'The development of a capacity for' is one of Winnicott's most characteristic formulations" (p. 488). We find the capacity to believe, capacity to be alone, capacity for concern, capacity for having a moral sense, capacity to tolerate anxieties, capacity for making reparation, capacity for confidence, capacity for gathering external factors into the area of the infant's omnipotence, capacity for experiencing unintegrated states, capacity for giving a signal, capacity for identifying with the patient, capacity to play, capacity to use objects and to recognize a patient's capacity to use objects.* More than Aristotelian potentials—with which Winnicott would surely have been familiar—these capacities had a developmental sense of the infant's or patient's possibility to meet the facilitating environment and become a unique

---

* Here he noted explicitly the developmental hermeneutic: The development of a capacity to use an object is another example of the maturational process as something that depends on a facilitating environment (Winnicott, 1969).

individual in the relational world. In Adam Phillips's (1988) words, "The emphasis on capacity ... allows for individual differences, [implies] stored possibility, [combines] the receptive and the generative, and blurs the boundary between activity and passivity" (p. 58).

In addition, meaning itself held a developmental sense for him:

> In [the] phase which is characterized by the essential existence of a holding environment, the "inherited potential" is becoming itself a "continuity of being." The alternative to being is reacting, and reacting interrupts being and annihilates. Being and annihilation are the two alternatives. The holding environment therefore has as its main function the reduction to a minimum of impingements to which the infant must react with resultant annihilation of personal being. Under favourable conditions the infant establishes a continuity of existence and then begins to develop the sophistications which make it possible for impingements to be gathered into the area of omnipotence. At this stage the word death has no possible application, and this makes the term death instinct unacceptable in describing the root of destructiveness. Death has no meaning until the arrival of hate and of the concept of the whole human person. (Winnicott, 1960, p. 591)

What something means—death or annihilation, for example—always concerns its developmental function and process. We should thus expect interpretation itself to be understood developmentally, and so we find it. Interpreting, no longer distant and intellectual even when filled with psychoanalytic words, in Winnicott's mouth sounds like rocking a baby or filling in his end of the squiggle game.

THE HERMENEUTICS OF REGRESSION AND DEPENDENCY

To meet the regressed patient without condescension or barely veiled contempt, leaving far behind shaming words like *childish*, *needy*, and *pathetic*—words they inflict so readily on themselves—we need an attitude and spirit already encountered in Ferenczi and Fromm-Reichmann's profound humanism, an attitude that forms part of the hermeneutics of trust. Winnicott found and maintained this attitude by linking his fascination with mothers and babies to his analytic work. Without a trace of reductionism, he was able to write that the crucial clinical question, shifting at every moment, was how old is the patient in the transference?* Without discounting his own contribution to whatever answer would come to this question, he meant that a developmental hermeneutic underlay every moment, hour, and year of his work.

Winnicott's clinical work, together with his long and absorbed observation of children,[†] convinced him that some patients, in order to recover, "regress to dependency" in analysis. Like Ferenczi, he believed that such patients need an analyst prepared to meet them, in Winnicott's terms, with "primary maternal preoccupation"; in Ferenczi's, with love; in mine, with the hermeneutics of compassion (Orange, 2006) and trust. But Winnicott, like anyone who works with the devastated, met the accusation that he simply wanted to avoid being accused of being a bad mother. He responded—nondefensively, I think, but from a developmental hermeneutic—to his own former analyst Joan Riviere:

> I think the misunderstanding ... comes from my pointing out that in the treatment of a severely regressed patient the analyst needs to adapt to the regression of the patient. It is easy to feel that I am saying that the analyst has to be a good mother if the patient is a small infant. What I really do say, however, is not that, but it is that in the transference situation when the patient is in the very early stages of infancy the analyst is in the role of the devoted mother. This is quite different from good mother. In fact it antedates a splitting of the good and bad mother. It pays tribute to the fact that at the beginning the infant is absolutely dependent on the devotion of a mother figure, without which the very early stages of emotional development cannot be made. (Rodman, 2003, p. 156)

---

* "One of the difficulties of our psycho-analytic technique is to know at any one moment how old a patient is in the transference relationship" (Winnicott, 1992, p. 181).
† Malcolm Gladwell (2008) thinks that to become a real expert at anything, one needs 10,000 hours of experience. Winnicott, according to several sources, had seen at least 60,000 infants and families before he began to write his important psychoanalytic papers.

His first crucial understanding, the one that removes him forever from the "school of suspicion," is that regression serves the search for the true self. The true self, and its emergence in a good-enough responsive maternal context, probably needs no introduction to my readers. Its individualist tonality, so incongruent with the rest of his work, probably belongs not only to Winnicott's personal psychology but also to the heritage of English romanticism, which I will later mention in considering illusion. This anomaly may account, in part, for his having confused developmental ruthlessness with professional recklessness in the case of Masud Khan and others (Rodman, 2003).

Nor does the false self need introduction, though it was probably an unfortunate choice of term for the protective system of self-abnegation developed to survive when "good-enough" support for unique individuality has gone missing. Arguably, however, it carries more weight for Winnicott even than the true self does:

> It is creative apperception more than anything else that makes the individual feel that life is worth living. Contrasted with this is a relationship to external reality which is one of compliance, the world and its details being recognized but only as something to be fitted in with or demanding adaptation. Compliance carries with it a sense of futility for the individual and is associated with the idea that nothing matters and that life is not worth living. In a tantalizing way many individuals have experienced just enough of creative living to recognize that for most of their time they are living uncreatively, as if caught up in the creativity of someone else, or of a machine. (Winnicott, 1971, p. 65)

It may be worth noting that the "compliance" of which Winnicott speaks refers to more than simple compromise or Piagetian accommodation that is part of all learning and life in a social world. Instead, like Brandchaft's "systems of pathological accommodation" to be examined later, compliance here means a life so profoundly lost that a radical restart is required:

> This second way of living in the world is recognized as illness in psychiatric terms. In some way or other our theory includes a

belief that living creatively is a healthy state, and that compliance is a sick basis of life. There is little doubt that the general attitude of our society and the philosophic attitude of the age in which we happen to live contribute to the view that we hold here and that we hold at the present time. We might not have held this view elsewhere and in another age. (1971, p. 65)

Given his view that profound and extensive compliance indicated acceptance of a sick half-life, we should not be surprised to find him understanding that some patients desperately need to make a second start. No prolonged vacation from the obligations of adulthood, instead a breakdown is an act of courage—a controversial claim even today. He also taught clinicians to notice the small breakdowns, just as Kohut did with fragmentations. Both understood them not as breakthroughs of primary process but as reactions to impingement or to failure of the needed environmental provision and support. Winnicott did warn us not to think "regression" every time we see "infantile" behavior or a few steps backward. For him, regression meant (and I use this word deliberately, as a hermeneutic indicator) an organized process of seeking a new start, more or less in Balint's (1968) sense of the "new beginning."*

Hand in hand, second, with his trust in breakdowns and regression as meaningful, came his respect for dependency and for clinical work that respects and trusts its developmental intention. Most clinicians will remember from their training, right next to the rules against gratification and self-disclosure, warnings against encouraging or even permitting dependency. Winnicott, on the contrary, would not have expected any significant work—with many patients—to be done without it. Here is an extended excerpt from a late paper in which he compared dependence in child care and in analysis, noting that most of

---

* Winnicott and Balint, Ferenczi's analysand and literary executor, pursued their studies of clinical regression separately, probably because Winnicott was so determined to work things out for himself (perhaps another aspect of his "true self" fidelity) that he even refused to read Ferenczi's work (Rodman, 2003).

us avoid starting new treatments just before we leave for summer vacations:

> A young woman patient had to wait for a few months before I could start, and then I could see her only once a week; then I gave her daily sessions just when I was due to go abroad for a month. The reaction to the analysis was positive and developments were rapid, and I found this independent young woman becoming, in her dreams, extremely dependent. In one dream she had a tortoise, but its shell was soft so that the animal was unprotected and would therefore certainly suffer. So in the dream she killed the tortoise to save it the intolerable pain that was coming to it. This was herself and indicated a suicide tendency, and it was to cure this tendency that she had come for treatment.
>
> The trouble was that she had not yet had time in her analysis to deal with reactions to my going away, and so she had this suicidal dream, and clinically she became physically ill, though in an obscure way. Before I went I just had time, but only just, to enable her to feel a connexion between the physical reaction and my going away. My going away reenacted a traumatic episode or series of episodes of her own babyhood. It was in one language as if I were holding her and then became preoccupied with some other matter so that she felt annihilated. This was her word for it. By killing herself she would gain control over being annihilated while dependent and vulnerable. In her healthy self and body, with all her strong urge to live, she has carried all her life the memory of having at some time had a total urge to die; and now the physical illness came as a localization in a bodily organ of this total urge to die. She felt helpless about this until I was able to interpret to her what was happening, whereupon she felt relief, and became able to let me go. Incidentally her physical illness became less of a threat and started to heal, partly of course because it was receiving appropriate treatment.
>
> If illustration were needed this might show the danger of underestimating transference dependence. The amazing thing is that an interpretation can bring about a change, and one can only assume that understanding in a deep way and interpreting at the right moment is a form of reliable adaptation. In this case, for instance, the patient became able to cope with my absence because she felt (at one level) that she was now not being annihilated, but in a positive way was being kept in existence by having a reality

as the object of my concern. A little later on, in more complete dependence, the verbal interpretation will not be enough, or may be dispensed with. (Winnicott, 1963, p. 339)

It is not possible to understand Winnicott's view of regression without reference to his underlying but rarely mentioned hermeneutics of developmental trauma. We must hear his key word, *impingement*, phenomenologically. In other words, what the environment does to interfere with, intrude upon, or hurt the baby's security may seem minimal to adults. Winnicott, on the other hand, always imagined himself into the situation and experience of the infant and thus understood ongoing impingement as devastating, as annihilation. In the original situation necessitating the regression in treatment, he described the following:

> It is axiomatic in these matters of maternal care of the holding variety that when things go well the infant has no means of knowing what is being properly provided and what is being prevented. On the other hand it is when things do not go well that the infant becomes aware, not of the failure of maternal care, but of the results, whatever they may be, of that failure; that is to say, the infant becomes aware of reacting to some impingement. As a result of success in maternal care there is built up in the infant a continuity of being which is the basis of ego strength; whereas the result of each failure in maternal care is that the continuity of being is interrupted by reactions to the consequences of that failure, with resultant ego-weakening. Such interruptions constitute annihilation, and are evidently associated with pain of psychotic quality and intensity. In the extreme case the infant exists only on the basis of a continuity of reactions to impingement and of recoveries from such reactions. This is in great contrast to the continuity of being which is my conception of ego strength. (Winnicott, 1960, p. 594)

He explained that in treatment "it is as if there is an expectation that favourable conditions may arise justifying regression and offering a new chance for forward development, that which was rendered impossible or difficult initially by environmental failure" (Winnicott, 1955, p. 17), and continued,

> It will be seen that I am considering the idea of regression within a highly organized ego-defence mechanism, one which involves the existence of a false self. In my patient this false self gradually became a "caretaker self," and only after some years could the caretaker self become handed over to the analyst, and the self surrender to the ego.
>
> One has to include in one's theory of the development of a human being the idea that it is normal and healthy for the individual to be able to defend the self against specific environmental failure by a *freezing of the failure situation.* (p. 18)

This may be a good place to stop and consider that "freezing of the failure situation" comes in a range of versions. We find encapsulated dissociations that allow for a life that is only periodically disrupted by retraumatizations, at least until some major loss or shock in adult life upsets the precarious equilibrium. We also find patients whose lives seem really double, competent and broken, just waiting to find the Ferenczi or Winnicott to give them "the advantages of a normal nursery." The frozen failure situation here may feel like teratoma, like a swallowed knife, like an endless darkness in which they try to grasp for a human hand and it keeps turning cold, and so on. Then there are Fromm-Reichmann's patients, whose failure situation has been frozen so profoundly that few, even in the mental health professions, can sustain a trust in their humanity.*

In each case the freezing creates dissociation, an inability to feel what is on the other side of whatever divides experience: self–other, true–false, teratoma–survivor. For Winnicott, the dissociative freezing protected a kernel of hope:

> Along with this goes an unconscious assumption (which can become a conscious hope) that opportunity will occur at a later date for a renewed experience in which the failure situation will be able to be unfrozen and re-experienced, with the individual in a regressed state, in an environment that is making adequate

---

* An extraordinary exception to this unfortunate generalization, George Atwood, has taught many of us to see the humanity in the most annihilated, to search for meaning where others pathologize, and to persevere.

> adaptation. The theory is here being put forward of regression as part of a healing process, in fact, a normal phenomenon that can properly be studied in the healthy person. In the very ill person there is but little hope of new opportunity. In the extreme case the therapist would need to go to the patient and actively present good mothering, an experience that could not have been expected by the patient. (Winnicott, 1955, p. 17)

Here the image of Fromm-Reichmann, sitting on the floor for three hours next to her patient who was covered only by a blanket, returns to mind. Similarly, we remember Lévinas: *hineni*.

Once again we must note, as in Ferenczi, Fromm-Reichmann, Kohut, and Brandchaft, that defenses receive respect and trust. It is normal and healthy to defend oneself in situations of extreme threat and to freeze the failure situation so that what is left of oneself may survive until rescue may possibly arrive. When disaster survivors arrive in a tent camp shivering and starving, we do not remove what clothing they have, but if we can, we wrap them in more blankets and offer them food and water and shelter. Our five hermeneuts of trust have all understood the traditional psychoanalytic attitudes toward defense and resistance as inhumane. Ferenczi and Winnicott, in particular, extended this understanding of human suffering to those who, when offered bits of hospitable understanding, allow themselves to feel and reveal how much more they need.

> The organization that makes regression useful has this quality distinct from the other defense organizations in that it carries with it the hope of a new opportunity for an unfreezing of the frozen situation and a chance for the environment, that is to say, the present-day environment, to make adequate though belated adaptation. (Winnicott, 1955, p. 20)

For a patient who needs regression, Winnicott thought, the analytic situation itself, with its inherent reliability, invites regression. If the analyst comes prepared to meet and understand and survive, the opportunity for unfreezing the traumatically frozen situation may really offer what I have called a "developmental second chance" (Orange, 1995). One of my most seriously traumatized patients has long described herself as "frozen," by the way, and many years before I knew that Winnicott had used this language. It strikes me, too, that Lévinas metaphorizes understanding as "blowing on the coals" of a text. People and texts need warmth to come to life, and the hermeneutics of trust provides this kind of hospitality and welcome to those frozen and terrified sufferers who fear they are losing their minds.

INTERPRETING THE DEEPEST TERROR

Winnicott (1974) taught us to recognize the "fear of breakdown"—defined just before his death as "the unthinkable state of affairs that underlies the defense organization" (p. 103)—as remembering earlier breakdowns, perhaps really severe:

> I contend that clinical fear of breakdown is *the fear of a breakdown that has already been experienced*. It is the fear of the original agony which caused the defence organization which the patient displays as an illness syndrome. ... Unless the therapist can work successfully on the basis that this detail is already a fact, the patient must go on fearing to find what is being compulsively looked for in the future. ... On the other hand, if the patient is ready for some kind of acceptance of this queer kind of truth, that what is not yet experienced did nevertheless happen in the past, then the way is open for the agony to be experienced in the transference, in reaction to the analyst's failures and mistakes. These latter can be dealt with by the patient in doses that are not excessive, and the patient can account for each technical failure of the analyst as counter-transference. (pp. 104–105)

Here is another example of the hermeneutics of trust. The annoyed or exhausted therapist could easily dismiss this patient, constantly looking for and criticizing the therapist's failures, as difficult or "borderline." Understanding that this patient suffers my misattunements as harbingers of psychological catastrophe, as indicators that the last hope of rescue from a bleak grayness where no one understands, may give me patience. Seeing this suffering may help me to trust that my patient struggles to hold on, to survive, to hope against hope that the breakdown originally suffered is not doomed to occur again now. At the same time the patient learns to realize that my failures to understand result from the complexities we call countertransference, not from the patient's badness or from some kind of inexorable fate.

Meanwhile, unfortunately, because we cannot protect the patient from this fear, temporality collapses:

> The purpose of this paper is to draw attention to the possibility that the breakdown has already happened, near the beginning of the individual's life. The patient needs to "remember" this but it is not possible to remember something that has not yet happened, and this thing of the past has not happened yet because the patient was not there for it to happen to. The only way to "remember" in this case is for the patient to experience this past thing for the first time in the present, that is to say, in the transference. This past and future thing then becomes a matter of the here and now, and becomes experienced by the patient for the first time. (Winnicott, 1974, p. 105)

This famous and stunning piece of Winnicottian hermeneutics gathers together most of what I have been trying to say about him: (a) that every understanding is developmental, (b) that the clinical situation remembers what cannot be recalled explicitly because it is too early, (c) that fears are remembrances,* and (d) that what sounds insane makes sense from the perspective of a hermeneutics of trust. What we have not begun to consider, and what Winnicott (1949) often considered, concerns the toll such work with dependent and terrified and suffering patients takes on the analyst willing to work with them.

---

* Terror as memory for me expresses the point so cogently explicated by Robert Stolorow (2007) that trauma destroys temporality.

A HERMENEUTICS OF COMPLEXITY

Winnicott's famous paradoxes constitute a central feature of his unusual hermeneutics. From childhood, he seems to have been acutely aware when the other side of an experience or idea went missing. Uncomfortable with his girl-self, he told Clare that he had set out to be more of a ("hating") boy (Neve, 1992) and seems to have incorporated this capacity to see and think otherwise into his life and work ever after. Dissatisfied with the excessively intrapsychic focus of psychoanalysis, he simply redirected our attention to the maternal system. Uneasy with abstract theorizing, he just abandoned it for descriptions of developmental and clinical experience that left the reader to find and imagine theory. Where others saw the baby, he saw the mother–infant system.* (Probably his most profound paradox, though not one that he so labeled, was to say repeatedly that there was no such thing as a baby; Turner, 2002.) Where others saw the patient's pathology, he saw in addition the analyst's failures. Where others saw delinquency, he saw attempts at damage repair and the reclaiming of what everyone needs. Where others saw a tattered blanket, he saw also a complex real and illusory experience on the road toward being creatively lived in the world. His own approach to interpreting everything throughout his life included this insistence on looking not just for the "both sides now" but for how these both sides work to create and sustain psychological life. Perhaps, if we could have engaged him in a phenomenological dialogue, he might have said that his paradoxes† constituted his manner of surmounting the traditional dualisms in which psychoanalytic thinking had been trapped. I might have been tempted to respond that these very paradoxes allowed him to avoid destruction of his psychoanalytic parents (Freud and Klein).

---

* Clare Winnicott said that he had seen 60,000 pediatric cases and always studied the whole family (Neve, 1992).
† Full of humor as he could be, he may also have thought of Gilbert and Sullivan's *Pirates of Penzance*: "A paradox, a paradox, a most ingenious paradox!"

In any case, let us consider in detail one famous, and one lesser known, example of his hermeneutics of paradox. The most famous, of course, comes in his discussion of transitional objects and transitional phenomena:

> The transitional object and the transitional phenomena start each human being off with what will always be important for them, i.e. a neutral area of experience which will not be challenged. Of the transitional object it can be said that it is a matter of agreement between us and the baby that we will never ask the question "Did you conceive of this or was it presented to you from without?" The important point is that no decision on this point is expected. The question is not to be formulated. (Winnicott, 1953, p. 95)

As I have written before (Frie & Orange, 2009), taking this point at face value and overextending it, we arrive at an absurd refusal to think seriously about anything. We throw up our hands and say, oh well, it's a paradox, or it's just an ongoing dialectic. Winnicott, on the contrary, took a strong position here, placing himself within the hermeneutics of trust. How so? He later wrote, "My contribution is to ask for a paradox to be accepted and tolerated and respected, and for it not to be resolved. By flight to split-off intellectual functioning it is possible to resolve the paradox, but the price of this is the loss of the value of the paradox itself" (Winnicott, 1971, p. xii). The capacity to live in the between—in the "potential space," in the transitional area, in the undecidable—means trusting the baby, the patient, and ourselves to find our way. It means trusting that we live in a common world (Dostal, 1987) within which not every problem (or gambit; Mitchell, 1986) needs to be confronted. It means holding ambiguity and holding complexity, so that our traumatized patients can have the chance to unfreeze.

The lesser known example bears a kinship to the "proximity" of Emmanuel Lévinas, which involves both nearness that cannot be evaded and infinite height or transcendence. Winnicott (1971) told a story of a boy who used string paradoxically both to join and to separate things and people and that neither function canceled out the other. He had to trust the child, the parents, and the

158 • The Suffering Stranger

emergence of meaning. The hermeneutics of paradox, I believe, expressed Winnicott's refusal of any reductionistic "it's this or it's that," his willingness to wait and see, and his sense of belonging to worlds of meaning. Within such a trusting hermeneutic he had no need to choose between embracing the process of making meaning together and rediscovering what had been long known, and perhaps feared, as in fear of breakdown.

This same spirit of embracing complexity infused his talk of "illusion."* Though always careful not to repudiate Freud, Winnicott deliberately contrasted his view of illusion with Freud's expressed in *The Future of an Illusion* (1928). Illusion, according to Freud, does not mean believing in falsehood or making mistakes. Nor must an illusion be necessarily false; instead, "we call a belief an illusion when a wish-fulfillment is a prominent factor in its motivation" (p. 31). We might say that Freud's Enlightenment rationalism, his contempt for what he regarded as religious self-deception and wishful thinking, met Winnicott's optimistic romanticism. Instead of wishful thinking to be unmasked in the "school of suspicion," Winnicott (1953) saw in illusion a developmental process unfolding:

> The mother, at the beginning, by almost 100 per cent adaptation affords the infant the opportunity for the illusion that her breast is part of the infant. It is, as it were, under magical control. The same can be said in terms of infant care in general, in the quiet times between excitements. Omnipotence is nearly a fact of experience. The mother's eventual task is gradually to disillusion the infant, but she has no hope of success unless at first she has been able to give sufficient opportunity for illusion.
>
> In another language, the breast is created by the infant over and over again out of the infant's capacity to love or (one can say) out of need. A subjective phenomenon develops in the baby which we call the mother's breast. The mother places the actual breast just there where the infant is ready to create, and at the right moment. (pp. 94–95)

---

* After I began to write this section, I discovered John Turner's (2002) splendid article, to which I am deeply indebted, but like Winnicott, I am unsure how much I have stolen.

Immediately we recognize the double, or paradoxical, situation of creation and discovery. What the infant, or the patient, or the creative adult generally creates, she or he must also find, and vice versa. The condition for the possibility of creativity, not only in infancy or in the arts but in every area of living (Winnicott, Winnicott, Shepherd, & Davis, 1986), is the between of illusion. For Winnicott, illusion referred to that "omnipotent" sense of possibility that fuels creative life, supported from the beginning by the maternal environment. In Turner's (2002) explication,

> The illusion of omnipotence nurtures in the undaunted infant a faith in the value of what it may bring forth out of its inner world; and its gradual apprehension of the mother's otherness fosters a trust in the outer world as a safe and interesting place in which to exercise that creative power. (p. 1072)

Illusion allows us to suspend worrying about what is real, because the environment supports us well enough.

> From birth therefore the human being is concerned with the problem of the relationship between what is objectively perceived and what is subjectively conceived of, and in the solution of this problem there is no health for the human being who has not been started off well enough by the mother. *The intermediate area to which I am referring is the area that is allowed to the infant between primary creativity and objective perception based on reality testing.* The transitional phenomena represent the early stages of the use of illusion, without which there is no meaning for the human being in the idea of a relationship with an object that is perceived by others as external to that being. (Winnicott, 1953, pp. 94–95)

At first reading this suggests a more pessimistic view than Winnicott intended—no health without a good-enough start—but he meant to clarify the basic relational conditions needed for a reasonably good trust in one's sense of oneself and one's world. Winnicott believed that the transitional space, or space of illusion he was describing, allowed the infant to develop this trust at his or her own pace.

> The mother's adaptation to the infant's needs, when good enough, gives the infant the illusion that there is an external reality that corresponds to the infant's own capacity to create. In other words, there is an overlap between what the mother supplies and what the child might conceive of ... [but there will be] an obvious problem on account of the fact that the mother's main task (next to providing opportunity for illusion) is disillusionment. This is preliminary to the task of weaning, and it also continues as one of the tasks of parents and educators. In other words, this matter of illusion is one which belongs inherently to human beings and which no individual finally solves for himself or herself, although a *theoretical* understanding of it may provide a *theoretical* solution. If things go well, in this gradual disillusionment process, the stage is set for the frustrations that we gather together under the word weaning. (Winnicott, 1953, p. 95)

Thus, this period of paradox and illusion form part of Winnicott's developmental hermeneutics of complexity, and the next step incorporates the inevitable disappointments and frustrations that come with weaning. The as-if-by-magic meeting of the infant's needs or fantasies yields to an increasingly mutual adaptation. Of course contemporary infant research has been showing that mutual adaptation and regulation occur from the beginning (Beebe & Lachmann, 2001), but Winnicott describes a recognizable developmental shift, visible also in clinical work, nonetheless.

In his later years the word *illusion*, with its rich allusion to play (*ludere*) and to creativity, dropped out of Winnicott's work,* perhaps because he feared misunderstanding and because he recognized the word itself as provocative in the context of the Anna Freud–Melanie Klein wars (Gabbard & Scarfone, 2002; Poland, 2001; Roazen, 2001a).

> I am therefore studying the substance of illusion, that which is allowed to the infant, and which in adult life is inherent in art and religion, and yet becomes the hallmark of madness when an adult puts too powerful a claim on the credulity of others, forcing them

---

* Meanwhile, a particularly creative use of Winnicott's idea appears in Slochower (1998).

to acknowledge a sharing of illusion that is not their own. We can share a respect for *illusory experience*, and if we wish we may collect together and form a group on the basis of the similarity of our illusory experiences. This is a natural root of grouping among human beings. (Winnicott, 1953, p. 90)

What I want to emphasize is that his use of *illusion* points to a trust in a dialogic and developmentally creative process (Tähkä, 2000) that relegates far to the background any form of psychoanalysis or psychotherapy that, in his words, relies on the "split-off intellectual functioning" characteristic of the school of suspicion. Again, John Turner (2002) said, "Illusion in his work does not constitute an alienation of the mind from reality; rather, it is the bridge between them" (p. 1073). As Usuelli* (1992) explained, the transitional space comes into being within the shared illusion maintained in the good-enough infant–environment system and, by implication, the patient–analyst system, for as long as needed. We hear no contempt or disparagement of "infantile" illusions; instead we find an embrace and welcome of the "potential space" for human creativity. In his review of Marion Milner's *On Not Being Able to Paint*, Winnicott wrote,

> What is illusion when seen from outside is not best described as illusion when seen from inside; for that fusion which occurs when the object is felt to be one with the dream, as in falling in love with someone or something, is, when seen from inside, a psychic reality for which the word illusion is inappropriate. For this is the process by which the inner becomes actualized in external form and as such becomes the basis, not only of internal perception, but also of all true perception of environment. Thus perception itself is seen as a creative process. (Winnicott, Winnicott, Shepherd, & Davis, 1989, pp. 391–392)

It goes without saying that, with Winnicott, we have left the realm of reified and localized mind: There is no localization of a

---

* Unfortunately Usuelli, apparently aware only of hermeneutics in the subjectivistic version of Spence (1982), expressed suspicion of hermeneutics as resource for psychoanalysis, at the same time as she provided rich and evocative literary examples of illusion that any good hermeneut would cherish!

mind self, and there is no thing that can be called mind (Winnicott, 1958b). Implicitly, therefore, Winnicott not only revolutionized psychoanalytic practice and attitudes, our focus here, but also challenged the underlying dualistic and mentalistic ontologies on which the more distant practices and therapeutic sensibilities had based themselves.

WINNICOTT AS CLINICIAN

Winnicott himself, perhaps to protect his patients, provided few examples of his actual clinical work and how it differed in practice from that of others in the British Psychoanalytic Society, so without the generous account provided after his death by Margaret Little (1990)—his patient who became his colleague and an important contributor in her own right—and the article by Harry Guntrip (1996), we would be left to guess about his work with adults. We know, of course, that he always worked with children, and he described this work in *Playing and Reality* (1971), as well as in *The Piggle* (1977).

Without going into detail, we can draw some conclusions: First, he allegedly worked in classical psychoanalytic fashion with neurotics (Little, 1990). If this were all he had done, however, we would not remember him! We can also say, second, that with all patients his style, including his office, seems to have been informal, unpretentious, and welcoming. Both process and general spirit embodied a two-person creative aliveness. His whole being seemed to invite the child or the adult patient into a squiggle play with him, in which both the difficulties and the hope of their resolution could come to life.

Third, with patients with "psychotic anxieties" he extended sessions, reduced fees, held the hands and heads of patients, did whatever seemed necessary for "management" of regression (Little, 1990). By "management" he meant taking full responsibility for the patient's psychological—and sometimes physical—safety and support, creating a "facilitating environment" until a patient could gradually take over more. Harry Guntrip (1996) described him as "more *revolutionary* in practice than in theory" (p. 742).

Fourth, he did not pretend to the patient that all this was easy for him, but neither did he rush the patient to recover quickly. He extended his normal limits with patients who needed this, but not infinitely (Little, 1990).* "The analyst who is meeting the needs of a patient who is reliving these very early stages in the transference undergoes similar changes of orientation; and the analyst, unlike the mother, needs to be aware of the sensitivity which develops in him or her in response to the patient's immaturity and dependence" (Winnicott, 1960, p. 594). Aided by his lifelong work with children, he often reached for understanding of preverbal traumatic anxieties and breakdowns (Guntrip, 1996).

A fifth clinical theme, *survival* (Goldman, 1998; Winnicott, 1969), is a complex idea best treated in my view by Emmanuel Ghent (1990), who shows how besieged can be Winnicott's version of the Lévinasian hostage to the suffering other. Ghent described *nonsurvival* as "retaliation, withdrawal, defensiveness in any of its forms, an overall change in attitude in the direction of suspiciousness [!] or diminished receptivity, and finally, a kind of crumbling, in the sense of losing one's capacity to function adequately as mother, or in the analytic setting, as analyst" (p. 123).†

---

* Writers like Kraemer (1996) have accused Winnicott, despite "Hate in the Countertransference," of neglecting the mother's subjectivity. Even if true, I think this is a serious misunderstanding of his project. As I read him, he was trying to encourage the analyst's care and caring for the patient in regression, and saw the closest analogy in the kind of generosity required of mothers during the period of "primary maternal preoccupation." Certain patients, he realized, would not survive with analysts too much preoccupied with their own subjectivity. They needed Lévinasians, people able and willing to realize a minimal subjectivity in their responsivity to the suffering other. Both Ferenczi and Winnicott came to think this situation needed to give way eventually to one that acknowledged the needs of the analyst too, and I would surely agree. But my subjectivity need not be at stake if I respond for a long time as a "maternal" psychoanalyst for one or more devastated patients. This, I think, was Winnicott's point.

† Had time permitted, this book would have included a chapter on the work of Emmanuel Ghent, another practitioner of the hermeneutics of trust, whose holding of complexity in theory and in practice I particularly cherish.

Survival, instead, has much to do with the analyst's self-care and with the capacity to communicate to our patients that they need not worry so much about taking care of us, parentified-child style. Jessica Benjamin (2010) wrote,

> To "survive" as a subject with externality means the analyst … assumes a reality independent of the patient's worrisome anxieties about having to be a caretaker for the analyst. [In this sense,] the analyst, being a subject in her own right, means she is one who can take care of herself and regulate herself … *not* an object to be omnipotently managed by a self-defined caretaker child who is desperately trying to suppress or regulate his own needs. (p. 247)

I commented (Orange, 2010) that we need in every situation to find our way to surviving without unnecessarily wounding the other or getting ahead of the patient's developmental capacities, as Winnicott himself noted in "Hate in the Countertransference" (1949). If we do not find a way to do what Benjamin described, then we end in the hell that Ghent depicted.

At best, however, as we noted in studying Ferenczi, working with the truly devastated changes us. In Winnicott's (1955) words,

> I have therefore had a unique experience even for an analyst. I cannot help being different from what I was before this analysis started. Non-analysts would not know the tremendous amount that this kind of experience of *one* patient can teach, but amongst analysts I can expect it to be fully understood that this one experience that I have had has tested psycho-analysis in a special way, and has taught me a great deal.
>
> The treatment and management of this case has called on everything that I possess as a human being, as a psycho-analyst, and as a pediatrician. I have had to make personal growth in the course of this treatment which was painful and which I would gladly have avoided. (pp. 17–18)

He left us with a final clinical paradox:

> What is it that may be enough for some of our patients to get well? In the end the patient uses the analyst's failures, often quite small ones, perhaps maneuvered by the patient, or the patient produces

delusional transference elements and we have to put up with being in a limited context misunderstood. The operative factor is that the patient now hates the analyst for the failure that originally came as an environmental factor, outside the infant's area of omnipotent control, but that is *now* staged in the transference.

So in the end we succeed by failing—failing the patient's way. (Winnicott, 1963, p. 344)

To me, success by way of failure sounds much like Lévinasian subjectivity through subjection—either a most ingenious paradox to be trusted or an experience of human finitude, or both.

THE HERMENEUTICS OF TRUST

How can we now summarize the elements of a hermeneutics of trust as they reveal themselves in the seriously playful Winnicott? Although he used "trust" developmentally, "the building up of confidence based on experience, in the area of maximal dependence, before the enjoyment and employment of separation and of independence" (1967, p. 372), we can assume that some such process underlies the clinical capacity for working from a hermeneutics of trust as we have described it in previous chapters. "As I look back over the papers that mark the development of my own thought and understanding I can see that my present interest in play in the relationship of trust that may develop between the baby and the mother was always a feature of my consultative technique" (1968, p. 596).

This sense of trust extended itself to psychoanalysis itself, at least as Winnicott understood and treasured it:

> The uniqueness of psycho-analysis as an instrument of research, as we know, lies in its capacity to discover the *unconscious* part of the mind and link it up with the conscious part and thus give us something like a full understanding of the individual who is in analysis. This is true even of the infant and the young child, though direct observation can tell us a great deal if we actually know how to look and what to look for. The proper procedure is obviously to get all we can both from observation and from analysis, and to let each help the other. (Winnicott, 1941, p. 240)

What was unusual in Winnicott's trust in psychoanalysis was that it included trust in the good will of the patient, just as Gadamer believed in the shared world of truth-seeking with his interlocutors. Symptoms, dreams, and regressions expressed the incommunicable, spoke the unspeakable, unfroze the traumatically frozen situations, if only the patient met a good-enough analyst, unafraid to trust the patient, the analyst, and the work and play of psychoanalysis.

For Winnicott himself, as we noticed previously, he first of all trusted illusion as a lifelong developmental and creative process. Again and again he reminded us not to suspect, unmask, or needlessly destroy the transitional realm of art, spirituality, culture as inherited tradition, and play, in childhood or adulthood, in life, or in clinical work. Instead, we therapists engage these illusory elements in creative and healing dialogue so that the child "in the transference" can have at last a chance to "share a respect for *illusory experience*" (1953, p. 90).

A second element of Winnicott's hermeneutics, also present in Ferenczi's awareness of the inevitable retraumatization of the patient, shows up in Winnicott, who believed that

> success in analysis must include the delusion of failure, the patient's reaction to the analysis as a failure. This paradox needs to be allowed. The analyst must be able to accept this role of failing analyst as he accepts all other roles that arise out of the patient's transference neuroses and psychoses. Many an analysis has failed at the end because the analyst could not allow a delusional failure, due to his personal need to prove the truth of psycho-analytic theory through the cure of the patient. (Winnicott et al., 1989, p. 216)

Once again Winnicott, like Ferenczi and Fromm-Reichmann, reminded us that our purpose, unlike that of researchers, is not theory confirmation. Nor should we expect to cure—too grandiose an expectancy for those who modestly devote themselves to the relief of suffering: "Psycho-analysis does not cure, though it is true that a patient may make use of psycho-analysis, and may achieve with adjunctive process a degree of integration and socialization and self-discovery which he would not or could not have achieved without it" (Winnicott et al., 1989, p. 216).

We can discern a third element of a trusting and generous hermeneutic within Winnicott's discussion of ruthlessness, a quality he attributed first to the baby's need to be met by maternal care that could also survive the demands of parenting (much like those of the besieged Lévinasian hostage). Winnicott biographer F. Robert Rodman (2003) wrote,

> The need is for one who will not retaliate, thereby fostering the sense of a world ready to receive one's instinctually based outpourings. Or, more likely, there is a range of needs, resulting from early experience and inherent temperament, which allows some to bypass permission-seeking and come forth with what presses for expression, while at the other end there are those who are on the brink of perishing for lack of a sign that self-expression is welcome. (p. 367)

There are many other examples in Winnicott of what I am calling the hermeneutics of trust: his view of delinquency as communication of early deprivation, his trust in the patient's creative capacity and desire to recover, and so on.

I do not believe, however, that it was the hermeneutics of trust that misled him. Instead, I think it was a combination of the hubris into which any of us can fall, with the cultural individualism that actually conflicted with his deeply relational theory. The search for the "true self," understood as complete independence, can make us lose sight of the face of the other. Or perhaps it can delude us into thinking ourselves capable of infinite response to the suffering other. The other's infinite demand on me for protection and care sometimes means that I must ask if I am the best one to treat this patient in this situation. Winnicott seems, at times, to have lost this question. Let us consider further.

READING WINNICOTT AGAINST WINNICOTT

It may be necessary to go beyond psychoanalysis. In the spirit of the younger Jürgen Habermas, who in 1953 read Heidegger against Heidegger,* we might consider the possibility of a double hermeneutic in reading Winnicott. We might wonder whether his true self, like Heidegger's authenticity, hides a dangerous valorization of hate, ruthlessness, and destruction, just as Heidegger used his "authenticity" and "resoluteness" to support identification with Hitlerism.

We cannot deny that Winnicott, most obviously but not only in the case of Masud Kahn (Hopkins, 1998; Kahr, 2003), allowed his spontaneity to get the better of his good judgment. Whether through grandiosity, hubris, generosity, or simple enthusiasm, he sometimes accepted patients whom many now, and sometimes he himself in retrospect, considered seriously unwise choices.

To my knowledge Winnicott did not write about the dangers his work involved. Nor can we deny that Heidegger became an active Nazi and never spoke out against their atrocities. The question, for readers and admirers of both (among whom I emphatically count myself), is how to refuse their mistakes and still see them as among the "greatest and fewest," to use the phrase of Emmanuel Lévinas (Lévinas & Robbins, 2001). Simon Critchley (Schürmann, Critchley, & Levine, 2008) suggested, for Heidegger, that we can find in *Being and Time* (1962) an "originary inauthenticity," an acceptance of our thrownness (our inherited situation) that places much less emphasis on standing out from the crowd and into the future as authentic. Critchley's version sounds to me much more like the minimal subjectivity of Lévinas (see Chapter 2), though his revised Heidegger would still be missing the ethical response to the face of the destitute other. Still, Critchley finds in Heidegger at least the possibility of a shared and vulnerable less-than-authentic life.

Similarly, I believe we could find in Winnicott—who of course wrote so much that one can find quite a range of things in him—the possibility of transcending the true self–false self

---

* Derrida (1978) developed this practice of "double reading" to a fine art, showing that the best reading of a thinker may sometimes undermine his or her own thought.

problematic generated in certain cultures and in particular family systems devoted to conformity but that may not be universal. Let us imagine a person, from a more or less disturbed family of a particular language and culture, living more or less his or her own life, within various forms of complex relatedness. Such a person, in childhood and adolescence, young and middle adulthood, early and later aging, will be more or less easily finding and articulating a personal idiom (Bollas, 1989). Relational contexts will evoke, throughout life, reactive aggressiveness, hate, and destructiveness, to a greater or lesser extent, depending on the meeting of actual needs that Winnicott taught us to see. I believe that his continued theoretical insistence on the indispensability of hate and ruthlessness as necessary to true self development is not only dangerous theorizing (à la Heidegger) but also a reflection of his personal psychology (Rodman, 2003). His family's requirement for conformity and niceness may have led him to the refusal of compliance and to the embrace of a theory of ruthlessness that leaves us with a more seductive, if less reified, version of Western individualism. In Neil Altman's (1998) words,

> Winnicott tried to deal with the ethical issues [of desire and responsibility for others] by deriving concern for others from his version of the Kleinian depressive position, which involves ruthlessness and love. Nevertheless, the legacy of individualism inherent in the idea of an interior "true self" remains a central, fertile, but also problematic, part of the Winnicottian tradition. (p. 947)

It seems to me that Altman has pinpointed an important source of the problems that Winnicott left us. Other sources of creativity—more emergent from relational experience and left unexplored—might have saved him and those he inspired from hubristic ethical disasters.

If, however, we return to the maternal* Winnicott, and in particular to "Hate in the Countertransference" (1949), we may find this "hate" as a feeling we can all recognize in ourselves when we feel overwhelmed by the needs of those who depend on us and resent them for impinging on whatever comfort we may have, as babies do on their mothers. What Winnicott advocates here is *not* ruthlessness or destruction but the acceptance of irreducible emotional complexity of love and hate, together with the parent's or analyst's responsibility to hold this complexity until the child or patient becomes ready to bear knowing about it.

> The analyst must be prepared to bear strain without expecting the patient to know anything about what he is doing, perhaps over a long period of time. To do this he must be easily aware of his own fear and hate. He is in the position of the mother of an infant unborn or newly born. Eventually, he ought to be able to tell his patient what he has been through on the patient's behalf, but an analysis may never get as far as this. There may be too little good experience in the patient's past to work on. (Winnicott, 1949, p. 72)

No saints as parents or as analysts or therapists, we wake up to care for our babies one more time, or to take one more phone call from a patient in terrible distress, without berating ourselves for our exhaustion or them for their needs. Winnicott gave us both the inspiration and the ideas needed to live up to our psychoanalytic vocation. He also, I think, did ruthless and destructive things that he could not see while engaged in theorizing ruthlessness and destruction.

---

* Readers may have noted the frequent appearance of the word *maternal* in Winnicott. Robert Rodman reported on his interview with Winnicott, "Freud himself [according to Winnicott] 'could not accept' the maternal in himself, because he was so strong a paternal head of his family. 'Yet the maternal is inextricably linked to the infantile.' And therefore Winnicott thought he could explain why Freud would have been personally blocked from adopting a less rationalistic approach to therapy. Freud could tolerate, indeed was 'attracted by,' his feminine side, as long as it was located outside in Sándor Ferenczi or other followers like him" (Roazen, 2001b, p. 177).

THE DANGERS OF HUBRIS

In ancient Greece, *hubris* described a person who, overestimating one's own importance and capacities, humiliated and mistreated others. In the classic instance, Achilles dragged the body of defeated Hector around the walls of Troy. In his *Poetics* (Aristotle, Benardete, & Davis, 2002), Aristotle explained that the tragic hero's flaw that led to his downfall was usually of this sort: A great talent, even a genius, becomes convinced that the limits and obligations that bind ordinary mortals do not apply. The hero becomes the measure of the right. The Greek tragedies as well as those of Shakespeare are full of well-known examples.

In philosophy, as noted previously, our worst example has been Martin Heidegger, whose capacity to see what was awry with the Western tradition since Descartes and Kant and Husserl intoxicated him and all those around him. Heidegger had developed a philosophy of the primacy of the situated human challenged to live unevasively in the face of one's own dying. He packed the lecture halls with students from all over Europe for 10 years even before he published *Being and Time*. But as his biographer (Safranski, 1998) noted, at some point in these years Heidegger became HEIDEGGER, at least in his own mind, and by the early 1930s had no doubt that there were no limits to his own importance. He hoped to be Hitler's philosopher, as Albert Speer was his architect, and as rector at Freiburg University (1933–1934), he used his own philosophy to betray everything that philosophers have ever stood for. (For an attempt to understand how this could have occurred, see Stolorow, Atwood, & Orange, 2010.) Here I consider him only as an instance of *hubris*.

In psychoanalysis we have many more examples, even among those whom we may most admire, beginning with Freud himself, whose ruthless excommunication of dissidents is common knowledge and who, along with Ferenczi and Jung, crossed boundaries of confidentiality that we would not accept violating today (Levine, 1994). Kohut apparently pretended not to be Jewish, as if he were important enough (or unsafe enough?) to justify such prevarication. Both Freud and Melanie Klein had the audacity to analyze family members. Countless therapists, beginning with Carl Jung, Ernest Jones, and Ferenczi, have become sexually involved with patients. Winnicott presumed that he could analyze friends and accept as a patient someone who was editing his publications (Rodman, 2003). Most of us could add horror stories that illustrate the destructiveness that results from flying with wings of Icarus (Mitchell, 1986).

Why do I recite this sordid history? Only to suggest that for all of us a temptation lurks, once we have rightly "thrown away the book" (Hoffman, 1994) and embraced psychoanalytic *phronesis* or practical wisdom (Orange, 1995), to feel dangerously expansive. This *hubris* can take various forms. Toward our colleagues, it can take the form of contempt or dismissiveness toward their work, where instead of explaining our disagreements clearly, we just refer to them as exemplifying positions with which we may differ.* At conferences, we can respond to colleagues in ways that humiliate and silence them for years and teach others to beware of speaking up. As Levine (1994) noted, "Most training centers have had one or more painfully recent cases of therapist-patient sexual involvement, and the problem of narcissistic appropriation of patients, often in the form of the cultivation of 'protégés' and 'disciples,' marks a thread of continuity between Khan's behavior and our own" (p. 1289). With patients, we may become far too sure of ourselves, even in our post-Freudian and relational and intersubjective "freedom," and create new kinds of iatrogenic disasters. Instead of blaming the patient for being "unanalyzable," we now

---

* I suppose that others do this too, but for the moment I will just note that I regret having done it myself, for example, saying, "Nor is it a search for objectively verifiable truth" (Hoffman, 1998) in my own work (Orange, 2002). It was completely misleading to suggest that Irwin Hoffman believed in the kind of "objectively verifiable truth" I was objecting to; indeed his whole project of dialectical constructivism goes the other way. I, like the hubristic characters I am talking about, got so caught up in making my own point that I failed to notice what I was even doing. And I have made this error elsewhere as well.

say, forgetting the asymmetry of responsibility, that we and the patient "coconstructed" the damage.

In short, I am pleading with myself and with all of us for what philosopher Charles Sanders Peirce called a "contrite fallibilism," a humble attitude that Sándor Ferenczi came in his last years to call sincerity. *Fallibilism*—a term Peirce invented to ridicule the doctrine of papal infallibility in the Catholic Church and to repudiate the Cartesian search for certainty, guaranteed by clear and distinct ideas—means a constant awareness that we can always be wrong, that there is always more to learn, that our understandings are never more than partial and tentative (Orange, 1995; Peirce, 1931). Without relinquishing our need to act decisively at times in practical matters, Peirce reminded us to "hold theory lightly." No matter how much we have come to understand, in part from standing on the shoulders of very fallible giants, we not only have no access to the God's eye view, even via Google Earth, but can really see very little and need others constantly to remind us of other viewpoints and to help us hold the endless complexity. Besides, as both Irwin Hoffman and Robert Stolorow are constantly reminding us, we live in the presence of our dying. This finitude means we are fundamentally limited, and so Aristotle had it right: *Hubris* is the big mistake.

Winnicott (1945) famously said, "We are poor indeed if we are only sane" (p. 139). Perhaps he thought we are also poor if we are only good. More likely, he thought that in the service of trying to be good enough, he could be a little careless. In spite of his blunders, to read Winnicott is to meet a creative genius who never to his dying day gave up on trying to respond wholeheartedly to suffering human beings, as the unique individual that he was, from a presumption that the other was trying to make sense. He surely embodied what I mean by the dialogic hermeneutics of trust.

6

Heinz Kohut
Glimpsing the Hidden Suffering

> *It is my great conviction that the most important issue in psychoanalysis is the empathic reconstruction of the interplay between the personalities of the parents and of the child.*
>
> —**Kohut**

Well-known to most psychoanalysts and many other psychotherapists for his revolutionary psychology of the self, Heinz Kohut has received less attention for his phenomenological hermeneutics, the reason for his inclusion in this book.* Because his self psychology is well-known and easy to access elsewhere in primary (Kohut, 1971, 1977; Kohut, Goldberg, & Stepansky, 1984; Kohut & Ornstein, 1978) and secondary sources (Siegel, 1996; Wolf, 1988), I will not summarize it here but turn immediately to his implicit hermeneutics. As my collaborators and I have written, his turn to a philosophy of experience in "Introspection, Empathy, and Psychoanalysis: An Examination of the Relationship Between Mode of Observation and Theory" (1959) marked a turning point from which he could not return. Much of his innovative

---

* Kohut's attitudes toward patients made it possible for me to become a psychoanalyst at a time when my philosophical studies, and my exposure to humanistic therapies, had already made me skeptical toward the orthodoxies of analytic theory and practice. Self psychologists close to Kohut whose understandings of him have influenced mine include in particular Anna and Paul Ornstein and Marian Tolpin.

thinking emerged in a contrast between attitudes of methodical truth-seeking, what he called "tool-and-method pride" (1975), and empathic values and attitudes. We shall see that the former often became apparent as our now-familiar hermeneutic of suspicion, whereas empathy, especially once understood relationally, changes the practitioner and the whole situation.* This chapter intends to show that even when the residues of older thinking—both instinct based and prephenomenological—remain in Kohut's later work, the hermeneutics of trust and his devotion to the care of the suffering other created a revolution in psychoanalytic thinking and practice.

LIFE AND WORK

Born in Vienna in 1913, and deeply educated in its intellectual and cultural life, especially in its music, Kohut fled Austria after the *Anschluss* as soon as he finished medical school in 1939. One of his fondest memories was of seeing Freud off at the train station as Freud escaped to London. Kohut made his way to Chicago, where he trained in psychoanalysis and became a renowned teacher and, ultimately, president of the American Psychoanalytic Association, friend of Anna Freud, and profoundly identified with the psychoanalytic establishment. So it cost him dearly to publish, even if couched in the old wineskins, the new wine of his phenomenologically informed psychology of the self. It is no wonder that he wrote so much about courage (Kohut, 1985). Many, if not most, of his older colleagues, including particularly Anna Freud, who called him "antipsychoanalytic" (Roazen, 2001b), shunned him, just as heretics and renegades had long been excommunicated from psychoanalytic circles. Even his followers, I think, have not always understood the philosophical underpinnings of the revolution he started, though they have surely understood his "genuinely

---

* Kohut acknowledged often that empathy in itself was neutral and could be put to terrible ends in the service of cruelty.

original spirit" (Roazen, 2001b, p. 141). I hope here to contribute something to clarifying this philosophical contribution.

His personal life, once he arrived in Chicago, was undramatic. He married Elizabeth Kohut, with whom he had a son, Thomas, now a distinguished historian. The autobiographical version of his emotional life, most of his colleagues and family believe, is told in his famous case history, "The Two Analyses of Mr. Z" (1979). Tragically, Kohut became seriously ill in the 1970s and died in 1981, at a point, I believe, when he seemed ready to take the implications of his own revolution further, especially in a relational direction (Orange, 2000).

His groundbreaking theoretical work involved rethinking the Freudian conception of narcissism without instinct theory. He had noticed an experiential fragility in patients generally considered untreatable by psychoanalysis, and he gradually developed his psychology of the self, which placed center stage in psychoanalysis the developing person in the context of parental support ("the selfobjects" because they supported the solidity, continuity, and positive valuation of the developing self). As a result, the classical view shuttled to the background as he asked, "Is it not the most significant dynamic-genetic feature of the Oedipus story that Oedipus was a rejected child?" (Kohut, 1982, p. 404).

KOHUT'S HERMENEUTICS

In his last years, Kohut sometimes said that he relied less and less on interpretation and more on reconstruction (Kohut, Tolpin, & Tolpin, 1996, p. 43). By this he seems to have meant that his understanding had become less and less based on preexisting psychoanalytic theory and more oriented to traumatic disruptions of development. Because we are discussing an inclusive conception of hermeneutics, oriented to all forms of understanding, it still seems to me more than appropriate to recognize him as a hermeneut and to note his belonging to the hermeneutics of trust along with the others we study here.

On the surface, it might seem that Kohut's hermeneutics most resembled those of the romantics (see Chapter 1), given his emphasis on empathy (Baker & Jones, 2008). We find in his works, however, no references to Schleiermacher or Dilthey or—on empathy—to Husserl or Edith Stein. Less surprising, given the psychoanalytic politics of his time, we find no references to Ferenczi's insistence on the centrality of empathic understanding.* As a native German speaker, however, he surely thought of *Einfuhlung* as feeling into the experience of the other. Unfortunately he often spoke of empathy as vicarious introspection (Kohut et al., 1984), leaving his early phenomenology just as Cartesian as Husserl's, as critics quickly noted (Greenberg & Mitchell, 1983; Stolorow, Atwood, & Orange, 1999). Over time, however, his view of empathy became complex and quite intersubjective:

> Empathy is so many things. Empathy is biological survival. Unless there's an empathic environment, a child does not survive. Empathy is emotional survival because, unless you have empathy in your surroundings, you feel you cannot show what you are and who you are. You know, in the beginning empathy is the reliability of the world, its predictability. Will responses be human? (Kohut et al., 1996, p. 28)

Kohut famously said of selfobject experience,† and implicitly of empathic understanding, that it functions like oxygen in emotional life. Without it, we gasp, struggle, panic, and finally collapse.

---

* Rachman (1997a, p. 355), however, quoted from Gedo (1996): "I received the commission for my 1967 Ferenczi article for *Psyche* through Heinz. He was my first reader and commented specifically about how odd he found it that candidates at that time no longer studied Ferenczi in detail. He was clearly thoroughly familiar with SF's contributions and esteemed them very highly. (He wrote me that [Karl] Abraham was Ferenczi's only equal among Freud's early adherents.) I certainly did not have to carry Those Coals to New Castle."

† Kohut used *selfobject* to designate the other used as support for the cohesiveness, continuity, and valuing of the self. He contrasted it with relating to the other as an object, psychoanalytic jargon for a real other person. The selfobject may not be experienced as separate from oneself.

> And if in an analysis you are empathic with your patient, don't expect that your empathy will be acceptable to the patient, to a disturbed patent, or without a great many problems for him and for you. It's your main tool, but it's also the major disturbance in narcissistic personality disorders. So, while you are so proud of the great capacity of yours, I think the angry patient, who has been so angered because he did not get what he was supposed to have gotten and now so needy and so angry that he has to get on his knees again to get it from somebody else, will reject your best efforts also. You have to take it for granted that you will be hurt too. You will be taken for granted. (Kohut et al., 1996, pp. 28–29)

This is the voice of a hermeneut clinician who understands how shaming the clinical situation can be. Hearing the injury and the shame behind the attacks and the protest is already hearing differently from the "school of suspicion."

He and Ferenczi also shared, though one must listen more carefully for it in Kohut, a hermeneutics of trauma. Behind the haughty and entitled narcissistic patient, Kohut (1972) could hear a tenuous and shattered other. He could ask how this fragmenting was reoccurring in the present with the analyst and what must have happened in the past to create such fragility. Although Kohut focused more on traumatic failure resulting from parental psychopathology than on abuse (Kohut et al., 1996, p. 117), his trauma theory echoed Ferenczi's in two important aspects.

First, both Kohut and Ferenczi saw empathic failure, by the parent or by the analyst, as traumatic (Rachman, 1997a). Empathic failure misinterprets. Just as we have seen the adult in Ferenczi's "Confusion of Tongues" interpret the child's attachment longings as a sexual invitation, Kohut's narcissistic parent mistakes the child's developmental longings as a refusal to care for a parent's needs or as simple inadequacy or badness in the child. Then, second, the traumatic effect deepens into a chronic traumatic state when the environment continues to overtax and undersupport the child. Here Kohut relies on a mix of older Freudian economic theory and his newer ideas:

> Such psychotic-like children ... are too full of disorganizing rage and destructiveness. In other words, they are in a chronic, recurrent traumatic state, chronic because of continuous influx of stimuli from a very, very unpredictable environment. And yet ... despite this over-stimulated, overburdened, overtaxed, and crazily acting psychic organization, despite it all the self is always able to reassemble itself once it is removed from this chaotic environment. (Kohut et al., 1996, p. 271)

He went on to describe what today we would call posttraumatic stress, and he called "pseudo-psychosis." He believed that both in childhood and in adulthood, such conditions were understandable and reversible.

Kohut approached the interpretive task in a simple, humane, and egalitarian way. He communicated, as did Harry Stack Sullivan and Frieda Fromm-Reichmann, that we are all more simply human than otherwise and, with Terentius, that if we are human, nothing human is alien to us. Patients, I suspect, recognized that they had found themselves with someone who would not condescend to them. Participation—a "we" sensibility—shows this attitude better than words describe it:

> In any normal human life narcissistic issues of triumph and defeat play a tremendous role. What kind of life would it be if this were not so? I find nothing wrong with it. We all want to be victorious. We all want to enhance our self-esteem. We all want to shine. As I said, there is a lot of hypocrisy about that. (Kohut et al., 1996, p. 73)

Kohut's hermeneutics, like all those that share in the school of trust, reject the tendency to shame and blame. Responding to the accusation that, having given up the drive theory that locates the source of patients' difficulties in themselves, he had become "the credulous victim of those of my patients who do not want to shoulder the responsibility for their symptoms, actions and attitudes but waste their time accusing others, including and par excellence their parents" (Kohut et al., 1984, p. 25), he wrote,

> The self psychologically informed psychoanalyst blames no one, neither the patient nor his parents. He identifies causal sequences,

he shows the patient that his feelings and reactions are explained by his experiences in early life, and he points out that, ultimately, his parents are not to blame since they are what they were because of the backgrounds that determined their own personality. The self psychologically informed psychoanalyst, therefore, with all the human warmth he may display, always remains a scientifically objective observer. (p. 25)

Though we may consider Kohut here to revert from his own phenomenology, his refusal to blame and to find fault removes him clearly from the "school of suspicion," that is, from among those who use unmasking disguises as their principal means of interpreting. Instead, he wanted to understand how hatred arose between the generations:

> These patients had parents who for reasons of their own could not respond maternally or paternally to them. And they began to hate their children, for their mere presence constituted a demand they could not fulfill. It is this hatred—which arises secondarily in the parents as a result of the narcissistic injury to which their children's demands expose them, that is, the recognition of their severely restricted responsiveness—that then becomes part and parcel of the severe self-rejection and guilt that the children internalize. (Kohut et al., 1996, pp. 201–202)

Kohut's insistence on complex relational causality reinforces his belonging to the school of trust. He thought many traditional interpretations actually exemplified *wild analysis* "because they are not based on the analyst's prolonged empathic immersion in the patient's associations* and do not proceed in accordance with the valid precept that ... interpretations must first focus on the psychological surface before they can move into the psychic depth and into the past" (Kohut et al., 1984, p. 93). In other words, we should take seriously the truth of what the patient actually said to us before we start seeking to unmask it, or begin searching for buried truth. The deepest truth, as Wittgenstein (1953) thought, may be right there.

---

* He does not say "in the patient's mind."

Although there is no evidence that Heinz Kohut had read philosopher Ludwig Wittgenstein (cf. Orange, 2009c), they surely shared a common phenomenological interest. Wittgenstein devoted much of the early part of his *Philosophical Investigations* (1953) to discussing St. Augustine's famous question and answer about time: "What then is time? If no one asks me, I know: if I wish to explain it to one that asketh, I know not." Among Wittgenstein's conclusions, which he thought also applied to psychoanalysis, was that we spend too much time looking for what is right before our eyes or what forms part of our everyday shared language and experience. Instead, he said, "It is, rather, of the essence of our investigation that we do not seek to learn anything new by it. We want to *understand* something that is already in plain view. For *this* is what we seem in some sense not to understand" (Wittgenstein, 1953, #89).* A few pages later we find, "We may not advance any kind of theory. There must not be anything hypothetical in our considerations. We must do away with all explanation, and description alone must take its place" (#109); "Nothing is hidden" (#435). Looking and listening together can bring truth out.

Trusting the truth to emerge in empathic dialogue makes this kind of hermeneutic deeply and humanistically fallibilistic. It brings a humility uncharacteristic of the theory and practice of the psychoanalytic tradition generally, it might be fair to say. But it is just this hermeneutics of trust that led Kohut to one of his most quoted sentences:

> If there is one lesson that I have learned during my life as an analyst, it is the lesson that what my patients tell me is likely to be true—that many times when I believed that I was right and my patients were wrong, it turned out, though often only after a prolonged search, that *my* rightness was superficial whereas *their* rightness was profound. (Kohut et al., 1984, pp. 94–95)

It deserves notice, I believe, that this sentence was not tossed off by the way but written like a testament, as if more than any detail

---

* Wittgenstein's *Philosophical Investigations* are always cited by remark number.

of self psychological theory, this is what Kohut wanted his readers to remember. It is perhaps the clearest statement in the psychoanalytic literature of a hermeneutics of trust.

In this spirit, Kohut began (and we will see that Bernard Brandchaft has taken this project much further) to rethink the psychoanalytic conceptions of defense and resistance. For example, taught by Miss F. who told him he was wrecking her analysis by interpreting (Kohut, 1971), he came to understand his patients to be protecting very fragile self-experience and realized that when they resisted his best efforts, he might well be doing something wrong that needed understanding and correcting. Only in dialogue with the patient could he learn what the trouble could be and what to do about it. But only within a hermeneutics of trust, and with an attitude that placed the need of the patient above his own desire to be in the right, could he have learned to question so deeply the "received view" (Kuhn, 1962) and to have found the courage to propose a new paradigm, even if one that in some ways would eventually need to be overtaken.

TEXTS

To get a feel for the paradigm shift in attitude and values that Kohut's work embodies, let us consider a few texts. Here, for example, Kohut was speaking to candidates at the Chicago Institute:

> I cannot stress enough that we must understand in real depth the meaning of that old technical rule that one begins from the surface. If it is just an empty rule, toss it into the wastebasket. You know, when you say, begin from the surface, [what] it really means is that over and over again, in each hour, you have to establish an empathic closeness with the patient, and until you have established it your best insights will be for naught. Now, obviously, in an ongoing transference, it won't take you long to know where you are. Sometimes you look at the patient and you know. But one still has to be careful. One doesn't necessarily trust one's first perception. The clue when you see him sitting there whether he's disheveled or well dressed, is the first smile—is it genuine, or isn't it?

> You know without knowing that you are in tune. This is where we were yesterday and this is where we are today. But the real issue is that whatever you transact with the patient must come from today, from now, before you get into the depth. Therefore—and I'm saying something very specific—the insight that people were deprived early in life, that they were unempathically treated, which is the broadest statement that one can make, is I think, the most profound statement that one can make about … people if one elaborates what this lack of empathy means. (Kohut et al., 1996, p. 22)

This paragraph tells us several things about Kohut as hermeneut. First and fundamentally, understanding depends on connection. There could be no understanding, and thus no useful interpretation, from a distance. Second, the empathic personal connection can never be taken for granted but must be refound every day and continually tended. I wonder if Kohut, who loved music, had in mind the need of a string quartet or an orchestra always to tune up before playing or even between pieces. Years before most of us were reading the developmental research and learning from Louis Sander (1988), Daniel Stern (1985), and Beatrice Beebe and Frank Lachmann (2001), Kohut taught us to notice the small facial changes. Furthermore, he warned us to hold our perceptions lightly, so we could notice our misattunements and be ready to hear our patients' protests. Above all, this very process would lead us to the deepest understanding of all, that for such a patient, attentive care had been missing* in the patient's early life. "Self psychology," he maintained, "holds that we can best understand psychoanalytic cure in analogy to successful early development" (Kohut et al., 1984, p. 152).

A second key text contains an incident that will be so familiar to readers who already know Kohut that they may want to skip it, but I include it at length for three reasons: (a) There may remain readers who still imagine that self psychologists simply affirm and support; (b) Kohut taught us to see and hear the suffering stranger behind the entitled "narcissist"; and (c) it may be important to

---

* A lack that may extend from impoverishment to Lévinasian destitution.

emphasize that the hermeneutics of trust may often mean taking risks to reach our patients:

> The analysand, who was in his third year of treatment with me, was a psychiatric resident at a university hospital where I occasionally give seminars on the theory and practice of psychotherapy. He arrived twenty-five minutes late to his analytic session. Entering the office, the door of which was open, he tossed his leather jacket on the chair and, hardly saying hello, tossed himself on the couch with a crash. He began at once to talk rapidly and related, with what seemed to me a trace of challenging arrogance, that he had once again been stopped for speeding on the expressway, that he had responded belligerently to an officer who had originally been inclined to let him off with a warning because he was a physician but who, undoubtedly amazed at my patient's provocative manner, ended up giving him an expensive ticket for driving well beyond the speed limit. The patient reported these events to me in an unrepentant, angry tone of voice, recalling similar incidents that had occurred over the years, before and during the analysis, including occasions when, while driving "like a bat out of hell," he had become involved in accidents—none of them of a very serious nature thus far. I listened to his outpouring in complete silence, but when after about five minutes, he stopped, I said to him in seemingly utter seriousness that I was going to give him the deepest interpretation he had so far received in his analysis. I could see his utter surprise at this announcement; it was totally different from anything I had ever said to him before. Then, after several seconds of silence, I said very firmly and with total seriousness: "you are a complete idiot." There was another second or so of silence, and then the patient burst into a warm and friendly laughter and relaxed visibly on the couch. I then spoke to him for a couple of minutes, expressing my concern about certain aspects of his behavior, especially his potentially destructive and self-destructive outburst of reckless driving, but also about other forms of tantrum-like behavior, including aggressive behavior at his place of work, when dealing with unresponsive salespeople, and the like. I ended by saying that we of course needed to understand what in his past, and, in particular what in his childhood, had made him so vulnerable in certain situations and led him to respond as he did, but first things came first: if he killed or injured himself in an accident, we certainly could not analyze his motivations. (Kohut et al., 1984, pp. 74–75)

They came to understand the sources of this young man's "narcissistic rage" not only in his original family but in a recent psychiatric seminar in which Kohut had apparently responded much more warmly to another resident's remarks than to those of his own patient.

Clearly Kohut did not intend this incident to portray his everyday practice.* He noted, "Confrontations should be used sparingly. They may shock the patient and momentarily enhance the analyst's self-esteem when he sees the patient taken by surprise, but they provide nothing that is not already provided by the realities of adult life" (p. 173). Nevertheless he clearly thought empathic practice sometimes included attunement to, understanding of, and appropriate meeting of dangerous grandiosity.

This suggests, once again, that empathy does not mean being nice; it means responding to the other's need as I am able to understand it in this moment—a more Lévinasian conception than Kohut usually gets credit for. In some instances, not to confront (or be confronted) is not to understand. In Gadamer's words, "When two people understand each other, this does mean that one person 'understands' the other. ... Openness to the other ... involves recognizing that I myself must accept some things that are against me" (Gadamer, Weinsheimer, & Marshall, 2004, p. 355). As a clinician, I must often accept my patient's confrontations of my mistakes, my assumptions, my hypocrisies. The patient, as in this road rage instance, must face the possibility that someone actually cares about him or her.

A third text, with my commentaries, follows a case vignette in which a patient, already fragile, developed psychotic-like symptoms after Kohut's long vacation:

> He had indeed felt overwhelmed by the traumatizations to which he was now exposed by virtue of his expanding activities, and he

---

* "On the whole," he said, "self psychologists tend to work in a more relaxed fashion, are more easygoing with their patients, have fewer misgivings about making themselves emotionally available to their patients if the need arises, and generally behave in a (comparatively speaking) less reserved manner than the majority of analysts" (Kohut et al., 1984, p. 81).

continued to react with prolonged intense suffering as a result of remaining broadly engaged with the world. What I had not seen, however, was that the patient had felt additionally traumatized by feeling that all these explanations on my part came only from the outside: that I did not fully feel what he felt, that I gave him words but not real understanding, and that I thereby repeated the essential trauma of his early life. (Kohut et al., 1984, p. 182)

Here again we see the two-part understanding of trauma and retraumatization that Kohut shared with Ferenczi. Something happens, but then the analyst's misunderstanding (as any explanation from a distance is bound to be) compounds the suffering and isolation. The confusion of tongues becomes frozen into despair.

To hammer away at the analysand's transference distortions brings no result; it only confirms the analysand's conviction that the analyst is as dogmatic, as utterly sure of himself, as walled off in the self-righteousness of a distorted view as the pathogenic parents (or other selfobject) had been. (p. 182)

Again we hear Ferenczi's plea for nondefensive sincerity in the analyst. What in my experience prevents me, here and now and with this patient, from staying close enough to understand from within the patient's perspective or from allowing the patient to bring me into his or her world of sorrow or confusion or devastation? Why am I leaving my patient so alone?

The task that the analyst faces ... is largely one of self scrutiny. ... Only the analyst's continuing sincere acceptance of the patient's reproaches as (psychologically) realistic followed by a prolonged (and ultimately successful) attempt to look into himself and remove the inner barriers that stand in the way of his empathic grasp of the patient, ultimately have a chance to turn the tide. And if some of my colleagues will say at this juncture that this is not analysis—so be it. My inclination is to respond with the old adage that they should get out of the kitchen if they cannot stand the heat. (pp. 182–183)

Kohut had long decided, with Ferenczi, Fromm-Reichmann, Winnicott, and Brandchaft, that dismissing so-called difficult patients as unanalyzable was an unacceptably easy way out. If some want to work with people who are reasonably well already, that's fine. If we want to work with the lost and the suffering, we will have to struggle with ourselves and suffer with our patients. Compassion means suffering with.

Here again we have seen Kohut's central hermeneutic principle: We must consistently attempt to understand from within the patient's unique perspective, without trying to fit the patient into our preformed or preconceived categories, diagnoses, and theories. This discipline, at least as demanding as the abstinence and neutrality required by classical analysis, requires attention to our own personal and cultural emotional convictions, the "prejudices" of Gadamerian hermeneutics. Even more, it reminds us that the Lévinasian responsiveness ethic sees reductionist objectifications, even those we have never noticed, as murderous. When we abandon this attentive clinical discipline, Kohut realized, our patients experience chaos and fragmentation. We see them disappear into dissociative states or dejection, or into confusion and desperation, right before our eyes:

> Under certain circumstances, when individuals come into the analytic session, you will see that they start right out talking about smells, but they don't just talk about smells. They will also be very sensitive. You know, you always move a little bit. If you write, your pen always scratches a little bit, and most of the time people don't hear it. They set it aside as one of the things, like thousands of other sensory impressions, they must ignore. However, now they come in and during the hour they smell the supposed mustiness of the office, or they have smelled a "peculiar, bitter smell" outside in the waiting room; and this also is the time when the slightest movement is a noise that becomes very, very annoying, when the sunlight coming though the blinds becomes very disturbing to them. (Kohut et al., 1996, p. 149)

Which of us has not had this experience, ourselves or with our patients? With the complexly traumatized, suddenly everything has become a trigger. What would have been a harmless remark or a shared joke last week has today become a minor or major clinical rupture, needing minutes to weeks of repair work. Items in my office or poorly chosen words set off retraumatizations. Kohut went on to describe the self-state dreams of fragmentation: "disorganized, chaotic, 'exploded' dreams like the disarticulated diagrams of mechanical contrivances that are purchased to be assembled at home—perhaps body parts or thought, or rapid, apparently incomprehensible content shifts from one section of a dream to the next" (Kohut et al., 1996, pp. 149–150). These worlds of fragmentation Kohut taught us to recognize as the fallout—"disintegration products," he often said—of unempathic human interactions, especially with us in treatment. My own guess would be that many patients become "unanalyzable" because they fragment under pressure from investigations in the school of suspicion.

On the other hand, as Kohut said in the Chicago Institute lectures, "Within certain limits, psychosis is in the mind of the observer. But if you can break through and understand something and build an empathic bridge, then the psychosis—at least that part of it you do understand—isn't a psychosis anymore" (p. 148).*

Here is how he might respond to the severe fragmentation: "I think you're feeling quite sensitive, quite injured by something, and it's too much for you to take today; something has gotten to you in an especially hurtful way" (p. 149). We can almost hear the gentle receptivity that recharacterizes whatever the patient says or does as meaningful, as communicative, and gives the patient the benefit of the doubt.

A final text illustrates Kohut's most famous—but also most hermeneutically significant—revision of psychoanalytic thinking in the direction of the school of trust and restoration, that is, his rethinking of narcissistic rage (Kohut, 1972). In general he saw what he called "free aggressivity" as serving healthy ambitions, not as manifesting an underlying death instinct. As for the

---

* My collaborator George Atwood has studied and described how this works out (Atwood, 2010; Stolorow, Atwood, & Orange, 2002; Orange, Atwood, & Stolorow, 1997; Stolorow, Atwood, & Brandchaft, 1987).

obviously destructive rages, "choking one's children, or kicking one's dog … violence on one's analyst" (Kohut et al., 1996, p. 107), he assumed that neither patient nor analyst approves but needs to understand that "underneath the ragefulness very often lies an inability to assert themselves. They break dishes and they choke and they shout and they smash furniture after they have not been able quietly and firmly to assert their demand for fear of how vulnerable they really are" (p. 107). To exemplify his theoretical revision, Kohut described a patient:

> He comes home from work; his wife picks him up 20 seconds late from the suburban station; he flies into the most terrific rage; he doesn't talk for hours afterwards. It's so obvious that he is in the wrong. She arrived only 20 seconds late. Previous analysis tried to show him that it was wrong to make such unreasonable demands. This analysis does not do that. How come? What else was there? How come these 20 seconds are symbolic of something so devastating? Is it really just a confusion of past and present? (p. 107)

Already we see the assumption that what seems unreasonable, even insane, carries meaning. These meanings relate not to instinctual drives or even to universal archetypes or anxieties but instead to a personal history of accumulated shame over ordinary human relational needs. These meanings emerge in the context of the patient's current life and also in the inevitable and painful disappointments in the analytic relationship.

> Your own mother worked all day long, and when you came home from school, you found a tired mother whose face did not light up, as if it was your right she would do that. And ah, yes the wife doesn't get dressed up. It isn't just that she is 20 seconds late, but that she's also not nicely dressed. She dresses only when there are better reasons for that than him. You know, he doesn't even know all these things. Her face is sour rather than lit up when she sees him. Then a whole host of meaningful conflicts rises to the surface now. For the first time he begins to say that he really understands how frustrated he felt when he came home as a kid and his mother's face did not light up, and the millions of other things. And only then can he begin

to assert himself and say, "Listen here, when you come, there is something—20 seconds is not late, but you know it makes such a difference to arrive here and see you waiting for me. That's really the difference. It isn't that 20 seconds is such a big thing in itself. It's that I come home and see that you are expecting me and that you have put yourself out for me; that you have put your dress on and the drinks are ready, showing that you are glad that I am back home again." ... I remember one patient who had a dream where he took a watch apart and he found inside the works why the watch wasn't running; because there was such a sensitive flower growing there. Behind all these rages, he is so sensitive and so scared really to show his needs and to assert them. (pp. 107–108)

Kohut—freely associating himself to the patient whose broken watch contained a sensitive but growing flower—taught us to hear the voice of the lonely, abandoned child in the rageful adult, a hermeneutic revolution if ever there was one.

A DEVELOPMENTAL HERMENEUTICS

Kohut once said, as we noted previously, that he had turned from interpreting to reconstructing. Though a shift from the school of suspicion to the hermeneutics of trust may not be immediately evident in these words, let us look further. To Kohut, understanding meant perceiving developmental processes that had evolved in the family environment, the emergence of the child in relation to the parents' personalities. Self psychologists, over the 25 years since the death of Heinz Kohut, have embraced infancy research and developmental studies more enthusiastically than has any other psychoanalytic group. This is unsurprising, given the developmental cast of Kohut's self psychology from its inception. Psychopathology was a sign of the failure of indispensable developmental/relational processes such as mirroring and idealization, and the psychoanalytic process consisted in the attempt to understand together in depth how the patient had coped with these failures. The conviction of psychoanalytic self psychology was that the very process of empathic understanding of the patient's life experience created the possibility of renewed development of a cohesive, temporally continuous, and positively toned sense of self, in short, a robust and resilient personality.

At this moment, developmentalists, especially the Boston Process of Change Study Group (hereafter the Boston Group), are offering psychoanalysis a new look at our clinical process. Engaging psychoanalysts of many stripes—classical, relational, and self psychological—their work is full of immediacy: the now moment, the present moment, implicit relational knowing, and working at the local level.* Let us concentrate on just one aspect, working at the local level, and compare it with what we think we know of Kohut's clinical practice. This comparison will allow us to consider once again what developmental perspectives contribute to a hermeneutics of trust.

Jeremy Nahum (2002) of the Boston Group described what they mean by "working at the local level":

> The split-second world of the local level is a level of small specific events, rather than primarily a level of verbalized meanings ... the observational methods of developmental research, which rely on repeated viewing of videotaped interactions between infants and their mothers, have illuminated a wealth of detail in the split-second microprocess. The minutiae of interaction, body language, gestural and facial expressive elements, vocal rhythms, tonal elements and timing can be observed and coded. For adult analytic patients, this meta-communicative or meta-content level is conveyed partially through the verbal medium, via nuances of word choice, timing, and prosody of speech. (p. 1052)

Clearly, a sensitivity to these micro elements of communication can help us to understand how empathic attunement, the gold mine of self psychology, works. Even better, we can come to appreciate

---

* Donald Braue (personal communication, September, 2010) noted that much of what gestalt therapy has always practiced is now entering psychoanalysis through these developmentalists.

how fine-grained our attunement needs to be, especially when we work with the kinds of patients to whom Heinz Kohut extended the reach of psychoanalysis. Best of all, we can become aware of what may be awry when things are going badly in a particular treatment and ask ourselves, in a Kohutian spirit—and, as I would also say, in an intersubjective spirit—what we are contributing to the misattunement, misunderstanding, or impasse.

Recently, for example, a painful bump occurred with a patient of many years, whose developmental history is one of psychological violence, betrayal, early parental loss, and methodical spirit-crushing without any real outside resource or mentor. Alicia was describing a dismal holiday season alone and proceeded to recount her long and complex story in a more despairing tone than usual. As I began to ask her practical questions about current plans and possibilities—not completely irrelevant but actually completely off track—I could feel her frustration rising. Finally she said, "You have to stay with me, as you have always done. I am not ready for those practical questions yet." I tried, for a few moments, to suggest that perhaps the continuing understanding and some practical steps could go on together, but the patient was having none of it. Just before the session ended, I told her that I knew she was right and that we would get back on track. But I was left with much to consider.

How could the Boston Group help me? If I could produce a second-by-second account of this session, or a videotape to be watched frame by frame and side by side, I feel sure that most observers would be able to tell me when the rupture began and to trace my chase-and-dodge behavior (Beebe, 2000; Beebe & Lachmann, 1988). It would be possible to describe the metacommunicative miscues in detail and then the lead-up to the moment when the patient told me to stop. It would also be possible that in retrospect we will consider this to have been a "now moment" that will deepen into a moment of meeting if we reflect on it together in the coming weeks. Again in the words of Nahum (2002), relying on the work of Pally and Olds, "In infant observational studies, this split-second world is where relational life happens. Although the therapeutic medium is linguistic, the interactions we observe here and patterns that emerge are largely implicit, in that *much of what transpires does not enter reflective consciousness"* (p. 1052, emphasis in original).

Another helpful emphasis of the Boston Group is on the inherent "sloppiness" of the therapeutic/analytic process, which probably contributes to what I have called fallibilism, or the error-proneness of understanding. Again in Nahum's words,

> No two partners can ever remain perfectly aligned in their interaction, nor would that necessarily be desirable. Since interaction is unscripted, poorly fitted interactions are inevitable. The interactants will go past each other. They will go away, come back, pause, indicate that they want things to continue or to change. The interactive process has many sources of "noise" or sloppiness that are part of the complexity of interaction. (p. 1055)

Because my patient and I share an interest in self-organizing systems, and neither of us really expects our process to be linear, at least not consciously, one might think we would just accept this as a moment of sloppiness and move on to increasing fittedness. But this is exactly where the "local-level" emphasis may leave us short. Such ruptures, in my view, though they are surely to be expected—even we hermeneuts believe that misunderstanding is indispensable to larger processes of understanding—have larger meanings not accessible from the local level.

By way of comparison and contrast, let us return for a moment to Kohut's clinical approach. Kohut's self psychology brought to center stage in our clinical thinking the importance of processes of rupture-and-repair, those very misattunements that can lead to increased dyadic fittedness so well studied by the Boston Group. For the first time in psychoanalytic history, Ferenczi aside, the analyst was encouraged to ask himself or herself what he or she had contributed to the misunderstanding and not to attribute ruptures solely to the patient's resistance to acknowledging the unconscious impulses.

There are, however, two important differences between Kohutian rupture-and-repair and developmentalists' misattunements (see also Beebe & Lachmann, 2001). First is the clearer recognition by the developmentalists that *both* partners are always working at the process of fitting together, not just the caregiver, parent, or therapist. Many of us have learned to hear our patient's protests, "you have to stay with me," not as attacks or resistances in the traditional sense of that term* but rather as the patient's participation in the process of creating understanding together—increasing fittedness, the Boston Group would say. Both partners are supporting and challenging the efforts of the other to connect.

Second, Kohutian rupture-and-repair occurs, at least apparently, at the macro level, as part of the larger life story of both participants and of the story emerging from their attempts at mutual understanding. Let us reconsider for a moment the road rage account. Kohut's immediate response concerned his patient's safety and that of others on the highway. Framing such a "nothing is hidden" interpretation as the deepest of the entire analysis opened the exploration of a wound between them that the patient had been ashamed to mention, his envy of the other resident's receiving the attentive reply from Kohut, the response he so much needed and desired. Kohut's capacity to hear nondefensively the way he had injured his patient—evidently, though he did not tell us this, out of his own performance blind spots that allowed him to forget his patient's vulnerabilities in that situation—allowed the wound between them to heal and opened the possibility of other sources of shame, underlying the narcissistic-rage outbursts, to come into the conversation. Such repairs require the participation of both and involve honesty and sincerity from both (Ferenczi & Dupont, 1988).

Kohut[†] insisted that psychoanalysis studies *complex* psychological states and that biologically based developmental processes can

---

* See Chapter 7 on Bernard Brandchaft for his further rethinking of defense and resistance.
† The following four paragraphs contain text borrowed from my book review essay (Orange, 2000).

be understood only in their emotional contexts. He thought that a child needs a parent "who responds not to isolated fragments of the child (drives), but is able to respond to the *whole* child" (Kohut et al., 1996, p. 206). A person is not a bundle of drives, symptoms, behaviors, or any other atomistic abstractions; a person, in Kohut's view, is a totality (e.g., Kohut et al., 1996, p. 249). In the Chicago Institute lectures, he spoke of the total or whole self, more often than the "nuclear self," an inclusive concept he derived from the experiential "sense of the completeness of ourselves" (p. 95).* He certainly thought that experience is always complex and requires organization: "I think that the experiences of the baby are compounds right from the beginning, albeit relatively simple ones; they are not isolated drives" (p. 198). And further, "Aggression, in particular, is from the beginning but one factor in an already complex psychological structure in which it is embedded" (p. 199). Most important, the parent's psychological organization forms the context of the child's development: "The child's self gradually develops within this matrix of maternal expectations" (p. 237). These refusals of mechanism, reduction, and atomism, in favor of complexity, holistic contextualism, and humanism, provide important clues, I believe, to the character and direction of Kohut's later thinking.

Kohut was extremely interested in the revolution within the philosophy of science made necessary by the theories of relativity and indeterminacy. Relativity and quantum physics had replaced Newtonian absolute space and time. Simple subject–object empiricism would no longer do. The observer and the observed were inextricably involved. But Kohut went further—and this

---

* This sense of self could easily include what relational theorists today call multiple selves (I think Kohut would be surprised to hear self psychology criticized in relational circles as too devoted to the unitary mind). In his words, "I have come across the possibility—at least I take it very seriously—that there are individuals, and perhaps many more than we realize, who indeed have a number of selves and it is not an illness, not split personalities. These individuals can draw on different cohesive formations of themselves that exist on the surface and in depth and are independent from one another" (Kohut et al., 1996, p. 76). Sometimes he spoke of self as "an important organizing center" (p. 190).

may be the key to his originality in psychoanalysis—to insist on a thorough-going psychology of experience as fundamental to psychoanalysis and psychoanalytic theory. He wanted to know how something *lives* in a person's experience, what it feels like to be in that emotional predicament, what is "the total situation in which the baby becomes enraged" (Kohut et al., 1996, p. 68). He was thus often impatient with diagnostic questions and refused to consider psychoanalytic concepts one at time: "Unless you take in the totality of a situation, a single definition becomes meaningless. Each definition has to be understood within the totality of a psychological experience" (p. 65). And again, "We deal with a psychological universe, with an introspectively and empathically grasped universe, and the abstractions are code words for that experienced psychological universe. In other words, I take psychologic life seriously as *psychologic* life" (p. 181).

Similarly, in teaching he was often impatient with a focus on clinical details or on specific pathologies and symptoms. He did not want to lose the forest for the trees. Let's look at the "broad, general significance," he might say. Or, for example, "perversions need an explanation in which broader aspects of the total personality are considered" (p. 3). A focus on experience is not the same as a focus on details. Kohut saw that the details of a person's life often become troublesome because of their emotional embeddedness in larger organizations and contexts of experience. He was always interested in the big picture, in the overwhelming character of emotionally problematic experience, in the "curve of life" (Wolf, 1997), and in the meaning of clinical details for psychoanalytic theory generally.

For this reason, he often cautioned students against jumping to conclusions, and he recommended staying attuned to complexity:

> The principle for all of you, as it is always for me, must remain the following: do not be swept away by an aha-closure when you have an insight, when you suddenly come to the conviction that you have understood something. Instead try to achieve other empathic closures; collect as many alternative explanations for a

clinical situation as will possibly fit. Then with the background of the various alternatives in mind, observe the clinical material afresh, over and over again. Observe the responses to trial interpretations, for example, or simply sit back and observe the further unrolling. (Kohut et al., 1996, pp. 206–207)

Here Kohut the hermeneut works the classic hermeneutic circle, back and forth between whole and parts, fallibilistically checking his hunches on the assumption that he could be wrong or less right than his patient.

Kohut was also a phenomenologist in his emphasis on time, process, history, and development. He resisted static, time-isolated concepts of anything. He distinguished, for example, between etiological (static, cause-and-effect) and genetic (developmental) points of view: "The fact that a particular child is lost at a particular time is not the etiology of his illness and yet, genetically, it's a very centrally located memory. It stands for the more personal feeling that I wasn't being paid attention to, I was allowed to get lost" (Kohut et al., 1996, p. 19). Although attending to misunderstandings in analysis, Kohut refused to isolate the here and now or even to keep it center stage. Once the misunderstanding is clarified, there is always a developmental trouble: "The insight that people were deprived early in life, that they were unempathically treated, which is the broadest statement that one can make, I think, the most profound statement one can make ... if one elaborates what this lack of empathy means" (p. 22).

So how might Kohut have commented on this not-ready-for-practical-questions moment in my work with Alicia? As interesting as he might have found the local-level focus of the Boston Group, my guess is that he would have looked for context, for the larger gestalt within which this occurrence makes sense, and for the relational conditions, early and proximate, that made the rupture possible and likely. He would have been interested in the trajectory toward increasing personal cohesion that Alicia felt had resulted from our work together and in what had made it possible. He might have noted that my implicit validation of the patient's personal experience had contributed to her greater trust in her own experience and would have attributed this to the mobilization and working through of a mirroring transference. This same validation might have made it possible for her to challenge me. He might have guessed that my leading questions had outstripped the patient's leading edge and left her feeling unaccompanied and unsupported by needed selfobject experience. He might further have speculated that my intentness on my own agenda recapitulated earlier attempts by important adults to dominate Alicia as a child and adolescent. In other words, he would have looked for multiple and larger contextual gestalts of meaning that made my patient's protest understandable.

In addition, if Heinz Kohut had been my supervisor, he would probably have asked what had led me away from my regular ways of being with this patient. A form of fallibilism appears at times in Kohut—the aspect that I have called perspectival realism (Orange, 1995) and to which other relational theorists allude when they speak of mutuality. I refer, for example, to his statement that "the analysis of the analyst by the patient is not a negligible thing" (Kohut et al., 1996, p. 14) and is not always the product of resistance. Kohut acknowledged that he had learned much about his own "narcissistic vulnerabilities" (his term in 1972) from his patients.* A readiness to learn about ourselves from our patients implies assuming we do not already know everything, that our own view can never be more than a perspective shaped and limited by our personal history and emotional convictions, and that a relational situation such as analysis may teach us things that can emerge only from the interplay and dialogue of different perspectives, of different worlds of experience. In addition, therapists must not hide, especially from ourselves, our hurt feelings when patients show us our flaws. Here are his surprisingly Ferenczian words:

---

* Whether Kohut had read Fromm-Reichmann's colleague Harold Searles (1975), I do not know; like Winnicott, he rarely acknowledged his sources.

> Saying all this [that attacks on the analyst do not necessarily have to be resistance and that we must find the meanings to patients of our disappointing them] does not mean that the analyst can never have any emotions, that the analyst must always be miles above human reaction and God-like in his understanding. That simply cannot be. It is much more important to realize one's frustrations, one's despair sometimes, the anger that is mobilized in oneself, and to realize as well the struggle in which these feelings are opposed by one's experience, one's sense of participating in an understandable process, one's ability, despite one's human reactions, to speak to the essentials of participating in the process. … I can see myself supervising people who set themselves on such a high throne, distant from what the patient does, that in a sense this kind of superiority and detachment is more of an attack on the patient than an honestly expressed annoyance. If you are so God-like and unattackable, you frustrate the patient even more. I think the only sensible way … is to voice an open struggle in the analyst's personality too. (Kohut et al., 1984, p. 99)

With Alicia, I became aware that from the beginning of the session, I had felt more pulled than usual into her sorrow and hopelessness, which also seemed more focal than usual. Because my own preferred way of coping with such feelings has always been to work, I went to work, concocting practical schemes. I forgot what this patient has been teaching me for years: to wait, to listen, to be there, and thus to affirm the patient's human dignity. Why did I forget? Most likely I had for several days been preoccupied with impending losses in my personal life, which in turn evoked living memories of past, extremely painful losses. Unwittingly, I then became the next threatened loss for my already loss-preoccupied patient. I became the next in a long line of humiliators to cast her down into shame over her personal needs and ways of being.

You can probably hear that my own reflections on this session have the more big-picture quality that I associate with Kohut and with the work of our intersubjective systems group. Still, I can quickly acknowledge that the entire rupture, as well as the probable repair, takes place also on the moment-to-moment "local level" and that attention to this level, if it cannot prevent such ruptures, can give us some hints about the elements that might go into resolving them. Such resolution may involve some explicit consideration of elements of the analytic work that had until now remained implicit*—mutual expectancies, for example.

What I conclude from comparing the Boston Group's emphasis on the "local level" with the Kohutian emphasis on the larger process is that both are indispensable and that they will shift in our clinical thinking like figure-and-ground. Clinicians, like people generally, will also vary, depending on their temperaments, their personal experience, and their theories, in their preference for the forest or the trees. Guided by the mantra that the whole is always more than the sum of the parts, I tend toward those who favor the forest. I imagine myself as an ensemble string player, for example, constantly attuning to the others in pitch and rhythm and tone color, but primarily attuned to the ongoingness of the music itself, another version of working the hermeneutic circle. With my patients, at most times, I try to remain close to their ongoing experience and to participate in its emergence. When discordance predominates, I become more aware of the "local level" and try to get back in tune with the ensemble so that the music can continue.

My preference for Kohut's emphasis on the forest over the trees also relates to the hermeneutics of trust. Though I take the Boston Group also to belong to the school of trust in general, it seems to me that giving the other the benefit of the doubt often depends on our keeping the whole developmental picture in mind, as both Kohut and Winnicott would have us do. On the other hand, both present-moment, local-level emphases and overall-developmental environment emphases support our attentive response to the suffering and devastated other.

---

* My use of the word *implicit* here clearly implies that I do not accept a radical dichotomy between the implicit and explicit realms of memory, perception, and knowing, as do those theorists who identify these realms strictly with localized right and left brain processes, respectively.

Among the less noticed but crucial features of Heinz Kohut's self psychology was his emphasis on the developmental necessity of disappointment. Though I have not found him to make this connection explicitly, for me this connects to his transition to the sense of the tragic in human life (Kohut, 1977). We are always deeply flawed and so are our parents and our heroes, starting with Freud and including all those we study in this book, even though I choose to concentrate on their contributions rather than on their serious mistakes. Their failings, defects, pathologies, even transgressions, like our own, can force us to limit our idealization of them and keep us seeking our own path and our own voice. If others' failings do not destroy us—this is the hope of psychoanalysis—then we have the hope of emerging from our shame without having to put our eyes out (like Oedipus) to avoid seeing them and can resume our life.

KOHUT AS PRACTITIONER OF THE HERMENEUTICS OF TRUST

Apart from the specific theories of his psychoanalytic self psychology, Heinz Kohut represents for me, as do Ferenczi, Fromm-Reichmann, Winnicott, and Brandchaft, the revolution from "school of suspicion" to the hermeneutics of trust and the ethics of Lévinas that place response to the suffering patient first. Some aspects of this ethical hermeneutics include the following.

Contextualism

Nothing gets interpreted by itself. We have noted Kohut's cautions against making premature closures and jumping to conclusions. My own experience suggests that anxiety in the face of retraumatization—the patient's and our own—can interfere with everything we have learned about attentiveness to the many nested contexts of family, culture, psychotherapy, and so on.

Complexity

Though empathic perception might penetrate right to the heart of the patient's trouble, understanding in depth for him always meant understanding the irreducible complexity of a person's history. Staying ready to consider his own contribution to every fragmentation opened a new world of clinical understanding that the title "self psychology" only begins to capture.

Humility

The philosopher C. S. Peirce called it a "contrite fallibilism." Here is Kohut's (1982) version:

> Introspection and empathy may misperceive the psychic reality we scrutinize (already on the level of data collection), either because we are guided by erroneous expectations, by misleading theories that distort our perception, or because we are not sufficiently conscientious and rigorous in immersing ourselves for protracted periods in the field of our observation. We must, in other words, be able to tolerate uncertainty and to postpone our closures. (p. 396)

Ethics of Humanism

Heinz Kohut's clinical sensibility, his hermeneutic understanding, was humanistic and ethical in this sense: His selfobject concept meant becoming oneself through connection to the other. There could be no isolated intrapsychic human, and why would we ever even want that? With all his respect for science, he knew the need for human warmth and connection:

> There is a story about one of the expeditions of our astronauts that has always touched me deeply. You may remember it well enough to spare me the task of checking on the accuracy of my recall concerning the details of the actual event that took place a few years ago. When, during one of the moon shots, a meteorite smashed part of the space capsule and seriously impaired the maneuverability of the craft, the astronauts, after having safely landed back on earth, reported that during the hours of gravest danger they had felt one paramount wish: if

they should have to perish, they wanted the capsule containing their bodies, however burned into dust, to return to earth. The greatest horror to them had been the thought that their remains would forever be circling in space, in crazily meaningless trajectories. I can well understand their feelings. And it is reassuring to me to know that these three human beings—they would undoubtedly consider themselves first and foremost as representatives of modern scientific technology—harbored as the expression of their ultimate deepest desire the wish to be symbolically reunited with the earth: the symbol of human meaning, human warmth, human contact, human experience. (1982, p. 397)

The human face says to me, as it said to Heinz Kohut, who therefore rethought psychoanalysis, You shall not allow me to die alone. Although I agree with those critics who think Kohut's theory of the self remained insufficiently relational, I believe his attention to selfhood was his transformational attempt to respond to the suffering strangers that psychoanalysis had been neglecting and to treat them within a hermeneutics of trust.

7

Bernard Brandchaft
Liberating the Incarcerated Spirit

> *But the mortallest enemy unto Knowledge, and that which hath done the greatest execution upon truth, hath been a peremptory adhesion unto Authority, and more especially, the establishing of our belief upon the dictates of Antiquity.*
>
> **—Sir Thomas Browne (1646), often quoted by Brandchaft**

> *It takes one to know one.*
>
> **—Anonymous***

Throughout this book we have traced a shift away from the hermeneutics of suspicion—attributed by Paul Ricoeur to Marx, Nietzsche, and especially Freud—toward a hermeneutics of trust in our response to the face of the suffering other. Freud had taught us to read every statement of a patient as meaning the opposite of what the person consciously intended to say, and he applied this method throughout his work. This attitude and practice became normal practice in psychoanalysis and in forms of psychotherapy influenced by psychoanalysis—much like the culture of unquestioned "normal science" described by Kuhn (1962).

By contrast, we find in 20th-century phenomenology and especially in the psychoanalysis of Bernard Brandchaft what Paul

---

* A taunt used in my childhood against bullies and evocatively employed by Bass (2001).

Ricoeur called a hermeneutics of faith and restoration of meaning. This project, in the spirit of Hans-Georg Gadamer, has renamed it the hermeneutics of trust. In such a hermeneutics, we approach the other or the text with the dialogic attitude that the other has something to teach us (Dostal, 1987; Gadamer & Silverman, 1991).* We look for what is genuine in the words of the other and seek to have our own horizons of meaning expanded. We expect to understand the other better and, through the other, ourselves. In addition we try to understand our shared world that we always already inhabit together. We learn together from the understandings and misunderstandings in the texts and myths of our cultures and of our everyday lives. Above all, we trust the other to teach us. As psychoanalysts, we rely on the patient to teach us about her or his suffering, as we search for meaning—both found and created—together. Whatever we have learned from the hermeneutics of suspicion becomes transformed because our attitude toward the other changes when we practice a hermeneutics of trust.

As in previous chapters, summarizing Brandchaft's ideas, especially including his precise contributions to intersubjective systems theory, is a task left to others. The new *Toward an Emancipatory Psychoanalysis: Brandchaft's Intersubjective Vision* (Brandchaft, Doctors, & Sorter, 2010) makes the content of his views now widely available; I introduce Brandchaft here precisely to clarify his position as practitioner of the hermeneutics of trust and respondent to the face of the suffering stranger.

LIFE AND WORK

Of the psychoanalysts we study in this book, only Brandchaft was my live teacher, but he spoke little of himself. For the minimal

---

* "The basic posture of anyone in the hermeneutical situation has profound implications for ethics and politics, inasmuch as this posture requires that one always be prepared that the other may be right. The ethic of this hermeneutic is an ethic of respect and trust that calls for solidarity" (Dostal, 2002, p. 32).

facts, we have the account provided for his recent book celebration in Los Angeles:

> Dr. Bernard Brandchaft was born in Dover, New Jersey, in 1916. He was an undergraduate at CCNY and the University of Chicago and received his medical degree from Louisiana School of Medicine in 1944. Dr. Brandchaft was in the general practice of medicine in Newark, NJ, for several years and a resident in psychiatry at Bellevue Hospital, New York City. In 1951, he joined the United States Public Health Services as Senior surgeon, stationed at the Bureau of Indian Affairs at the Intermountain School, Brigham City, Utah. Dr. Brandchaft trained in psychoanalysis at the Los Angeles Institute from 1952–1956 and was appointed Training and supervising Analyst at the Institute in 1960. He received the teacher of the year award for three consecutive years. In 1962 he was made Assistant Professor of psychiatry, UCLA School of Medicine, Department of Psychiatry; and later an emeritus faculty member at the same school. Dr. Brandchaft is a distinguished Life Fellow of the American Psychiatric Association. He is a member of the Core Faculty at the Institute for the Psychoanalytic Study of Subjectivity, NYC. Dr. Brandchaft has taught and lectured in Auckland, New Zealand; Sydney, Australia; Rio de Janeiro, Brazil; and Toronto, Canada; and has lectured widely in the United States. He has published multiple papers and is the co-author with George Atwood and Robert Stolorow of *Psychoanalytic Treatment: An Intersubjective Approach* (1987); and *The Intersubjective Perspective* (1994). He was married in 1942 to Elaine Meyers; they have three daughters, three sons-in-law and four grandchildren. (Institute for Contemporary Psychoanalysis, 2010)

This dry-as-dust account needs some hermeneutics! It sounds like a long life, a distinguished life in medicine and psychoanalysis, that began about 15 miles from where I am now writing about him and is culminating in Southern California. To give life to this extraordinary journey, let us consult Brandchaft's own intellectual autobiography (Brandchaft et al., 2010). He began as a "normal" American psychoanalyst and later became deeply involved with object relations psychoanalysis—even spending time in England to work and study with such major contributors as Winnicott and becoming close friends with Wilfred Bion and Herbert Rosenfeld. Later he understood the importance and then the limitations of Kohutian self psychology and worked with intersubjective systems theorists Robert Stolorow and George Atwood. Reading his own account reminds me of why I long ago called him my favorite fallibilist (Orange, 1995): Each time, over 60 years, that he tentatively embraced a new set of ideas in psychoanalysis, he kept searching as soon as he clearly saw that neither he nor a particular theory's best advocates could resolve its internal contradictions, mitigate its negative impacts in clinical situations, or account for its inability to theorize his clinical experience. At every juncture, when he has clearly seen what his clinical work was teaching him, he has searched for the next step. This fallibilism may sound like a simple intellectual honesty, but as he recounts, it cost him dearly in personal friendships and in worlds of psychoanalytic belonging. As we have seen before with Ferenczi, Winnicott, and Kohut, the psychoanalytic world has always punished dissidents harshly. Although he has also at times seemed impatient with those who could not see what he sees, Brandchaft has paid for his refusal to stifle his own voice—as he sees it, the voice of those who cannot speak for themselves.

Brandchaft begins his own life story, evocatively, with his adolescent wanderings in the Great Depression that brought him to meet the kinds of people who would engage his compassionate determination in his later life as a psychoanalyst. Already we can hear his characteristic voice:

> I remember ... how my curiosity took me, in the summers of 15th and 16th years, to the roads and to the rails, freight cars, and hobo jungles of the 1930s America where I encountered whole families of dispossessed and solitary souls all lost in a culture in which alienation had become institutionalized. But the avalanche of history did not stop there. Following the Great Depression and the Second World War ... the story of my professional career is thus intertwined with a background context of a culture increasingly torn apart by a succession of traumatic events ... [in a] society ... in which no one was answerable and

every sector was desperately in need of fresh understanding. (Brandchaft et al., 2010, pp. 9–10)

He went on to say that psychoanalysis, in the grip of a doctrine of intrapsychic determinism, also desperately needed fresh understanding. His own journey, from ego psychology through object relations and self psychology, eventually involved him with Atwood and Stolorow in the creation of intersubjective systems theory, according to which patient and analyst, like child and caregiver, form an inextricable psychological field or system, outside of which no understanding is possible and from which no fully independent existence can be described.* Brandchaft described this collaboration as an extension of Winnicott's realization that "there is no such thing as an infant" (Doctors, 2010).

His entire professional life has extended both his adolescent curiosity and an ever-stronger determination to find and create sources of the needed understanding. Like our other reluctant renegades, Brandchaft has responded to the suffering of patients considered untreatable by most analysts and psychotherapists. In an era that idealizes the quick fix for every problem, Brandchaft epitomizes the marathoner (cf. the person with "intractable depression" with whom he worked at least for 17 years; Brandchaft, 1988), not the sprinter. If he finds the road blocked, he tries to understand why and whether he himself may be blocking the road with his preconceived ideas. This is an informal way of talking about his hermeneutics of resistance and defense.

THE HERMENEUTICS OF DEFENSE AND RESISTANCE

To me, an outstanding example of this type of hermeneutics comes into view in Brandchaft's attitude toward defense and resistance in psychoanalysis. Many of us had already learned from Heinz Kohut to understand defense as the attempt to protect fragile

---

* Other relational psychoanalysts use 'intersubjectivity' rather differently, but these meanings do not conflict, in my view.

self-experience from further fragmentation and traumatic devastation. But when I heard Bernie Brandchaft say—I cannot remember exactly when—that resistance is the attitude of heroes in the face of oppression,* I knew that I was in a new psychoanalytic world. Resistance no longer meant that the patient attempted, through cowardice, to evade and cover up base motivations and crimes. Nor did it mean only the protection of a fragile self against fragmentation. Instead, our patients were fighting for their own psychological survival yet repeatedly collapsing when we analysts seemed to require that they comply and collude with us in their own destruction or imprisonment. Therapists needed to trust patients to guide us to understand the oppressive situations that had necessitated these heroic resistances that looked like negative therapeutic reactions (Brandchaft, 1983).† Furthermore, we needed to trust that in a dialogic, hermeneutic field of psychoanalysis or psychotherapy, patient and therapist might find a way together to engage the struggle against self-destroying compliance that involved so much more than behavioral conformity.

Let us turn to Brandchaft's own writings on defense and resistance. Twenty-five years ago he noted that Freud saw "the patient's refusal to accept the analyst's perception of [the patient's] reality ... as the most tenacious of resistances" (1985, p. 90). This made the patient "the enemy of his own recovery" in Freud's eyes. Brandchaft continued, "Discounted was the patient's own perception of the reality of a fragile self and a tenuously maintained organization of self experience" (p. 90). Freud's account (what I am calling the hermeneutics of suspicion) included reference, Brandchaft went on, to putative adhesiveness of the libido, depletion of plasticity, need to fail, need to suffer, and so on. No wonder the discouraged and defeated patient, feeling relentlessly misunderstood, finally wandered away from analysis.

---

* Note later that he also said things like this in print.
† In a similar vein, Lynne Jacobs (2010) said, "What we call resistances are more like forgotten allies representative of the patient's strivings for dignity and selfhood in difficult conditions." (p. 2)

Even in the 1980s, Brandchaft noted, new forms of suspicion predominated: splitting, projective identification, pathological envy, absence of object constancy, and so on. The newer theories viewed the patient as constructing these defenses and resistances to protect—so the story went—from awareness of the true and fundamental problem: innate and disavowed destructive aggression.

Brandchaft's intersubjective psychoanalysis, on the contrary, proceeds on the basis of very different assumptions, some of which are held in common with those of self psychology. First, it assumes that "all intrapsychic phenomena are codetermined" (1985, p. 92). Whatever defenses and resistances occur in treatment result from the contributions of *two people*. Second, this means that careful attempts to understand what *both* have contributed to any misunderstanding will advance the therapeutic process. Third, with Kohut, we must assume that *both people* are attempting to protect and develop self-experience. Brandchaft quoted Kohut: "[The analyst becomes frustrated] at seeing his help rejected … and being narcissistically wounded, we tend to become enraged and then to rationalize our counter attack in scientific, moral, or most frequently, morally tinged scientific terms" (p. 92). We then say, in the most disparaging tone, that the patient is defending or resisting. If the patient is also a clinician, especially a training analysand, she may say, full of shame, "I'm so sorry for resisting." We can already see in the patient's self-subjugating reaction that she "knows" she must resist her own needed resistances (i.e., she must submit to the psychoanalytic system).

We can already see in this "resistance against resistance" the kernel of Brandchaft's later great work on what he would come to call the "structures of pathological accommodation," that is, the internalized requirement to give up one's own path to protect the absolutely needed attachment bond, in this case to the analytic community. The young analyst must comply without question with whatever standard of analysis the institute requires and approves or be branded defensive and "resistant."* This internalized requirement to give up one's own path, even of heroic resistance, to protect the absolutely needed attachment bond is likely to be repeated in analysis unless the analyst becomes aware enough of supporting the imprisoning demand. Brandchaft (1985) commented, with heavy irony,

> How unfortunate that psychoanalysis has taken over a term [*resistance*] for these presumed pathological reactions that in everyday language is used to describe the sometimes courageous measure taken by heroes in pursuit of the right to determine their own fate! How constricting that fresh generations of psychoanalysts continue to subscribe to the principle of "intentionality"—if they are frustrated and defeated that that is the intention of the patient and motive for resistance. When a patient feels frustrated and believes that that is the analyst's intention, it is clearly recognizable that the patient has failed, in the experience, to attain the level of development at which he could recognize the analyst as an independent center of initiative, that *post hoc propter hoc non est*! (p. 93)

To translate, *after this, does not mean because of this*! To translate the patient's frustration into the patient's "developmental failure" to recognize the analyst is, Brandchaft thinks, a cruel reversal. Sometimes protest and resistance are in the service of therapeutics and justice, but only a hermeneutics of trust like that practiced by Brandchaft can allow us to hear our patients' protests in this way.

Understanding that rebellion can protect a very fragile shard of remaining self-experience, Brandchaft draws special attention to those actions especially irritating to working clinicians—skipping

---

* I remember well being branded a "troublemaker"—even in an institute that intended to be less bound to the "dictates of Antiquity" than others—for asking why things must be done as they had always been done. In one instance, I had applied to the six founding faculty—which included Brandchaft—for an exception to training analysis regulations to be made for me, because of financial distress and because my training analyst and I thought we had done most of the work before my "training" started. When my request was refused on the grounds that rules must prevail, Brandchaft, who did not know me personally at the time, immediately sent me a handwritten note, which I still treasure, saying that he was sure the decision should be left to me and to my analyst.

sessions, coming late, not paying, and so on—and teaches those who would learn to work intersubjectively to give them careful attention as self-protective devices. He described his work with Martin, who regularly arrived late and then reacted furiously to every impingement:

> The most difficult problems posed for me involved sorting out my own reactions and their impact on Martin. This was especially exacting because Martin had developed an unusual acuity of perception, especially for dissonant, unattuned, or misattuned responses, and a directness and intensity of expression that were equally unusual. ... He was firmly convinced that the price of a harmonious tie to the analyst would be submission to the analyst, a betrayal of his trust by the analyst, and abandonment of his own strivings for individualized selfhood. It was threats such as these that had compelled him to limit, control, or withdraw from every previous relationship. This solution had left him feeling alienated and alone, endowing every achievement with an unbearable hollowness and every victory with a growing sense of empty isolation. (Brandchaft et al., 2010, pp. 81–82)

Martin and other patients gradually taught Brandchaft that their deepest despair within their treatment occurred in a complex response to his own failures. Once, Brandchaft asked Martin if he didn't think, given that he hated being kept waiting himself, that he was somewhat inconsiderate toward his analyst. Martin exploded:

> Listen. If you are asking if I am upset about being late, the answer is yes. And if you are pissed off with me, tell me so and don't pretend that what you are doing is part of the analysis. I have lived all my life with people being pissed off with me and then saying they are not and that it is for my own good! What I don't understand and don't like in you is not that you are upset but your subterfuge. (p. 82)

Like Ferenczi, Fromm-Reichmann, and Kohut, he learned that honesty with oneself and sincerity with the patient—I might say with Peirce a "contrite fallibilism"—becomes the absolutely necessary condition for finding the way forward:

> Even in those instances in which Martin's lateness could definitely be linked to some experience of misattunement in the preceding session, it was neither the earlier asynchrony nor the lateness, nor any other reaction on Martin's part, that resulted in serious disjunction. Rather is was invariably a *subsequent* failure on my part to connect empathically with Martins dysphoric state of mind, and to appreciate the impact of the prior misattunement on Martin's sense of self and on his hopes for himself, that would lead to a marked increase in his guardedness and avoidance behavior and to a feeling of unending despair. (p. 83)

The power differential in the analytic situation may often dispose patients to rebel against our expectations of compliance. Equipped with a hermeneutics of trust, we may begin to understand how they have been crushed and that they are beginning to stand up for themselves. Brandchaft's later papers are full of stories in which careful, nonjudgmental, and sustained empathic inquiry into the meaning of such "resistances" formed the central work of an entire analysis. They become, without replacing dreams, the "royal road" to the prereflective unconscious where brutal emotional convictions, or organizing principles, still hold their terrible grip. These convictions claim that if I choose for myself, or if I do not submit to your humiliating demands, you will abandon me, or shun me, or despise me. I will be finally and forever alone, even subhuman.

What Brandchaft came to understand, as he clearly explained in "To Free the Spirit From Its Cell" (1993), was that supplying what our patients had lacked developmentally—mirroring, the idealizable parent, the holding environment—would never suffice. These dreadful convictions structure the whole existence of a human being that has been taken over by the agenda of others at the most basic level, and they function entirely involuntarily at a subcognitive level, as portrayed, for example, in Gus Van Sant's film *Good Will Hunting*, in which the Matt Damon character resembles the most belligerent of Brandchaft's patients. No amount of interpretation, or of mirroring, or of gentle provision could reach the soul of a person so destroyed. Only the determined grappling, *mano a mano,* as Brandchaft often says, with the powers of evil can connect and affirm the right to resistance.

Not that we should intentionally deprive or frustrate our patients; working intersubjectively requires no return to "do not gratify." Instead, noticing the emotional shifts from self-possessed vitality to deflated hopelessness can teach us that there is no return to the beginning. Our patients come to us hoping for an attachment that will permit them to own their own lives, but instead they repeatedly find that they must give themselves up for their attachment to us. Finely attuned to every indication that we are disappointed in their progress, to our own sense of failure, or to our particular agenda for them, patients find themselves once again "imprisoned in the gulag" not only of their own minds but of the analytic relationship. Only when we become aware enough of our countertransference participation in their continued incarceration can they gradually become free in an "emancipatory psychoanalysis" (Robert Stolorow's apt phrase). In Brandchaft's (1991) own words, "This aspect of the therapeutic process, in my experience, specifically promotes the development in the patient of an independent center of initiative and a sustaining enthusiasm for an evolving design that expresses the patient's own distinctness" (p. 105).

THE HERMENEUTICS OF INTERSUBJECTIVITY

Not for nothing was Bernard Brandchaft the collaborator, perhaps even at moments the catalyst, with Atwood and Stolorow in the development of intersubjective systems theory. This theory* sees

---

* Brandchaft was involved in its development almost from the beginning (Atwood & Stolorow, 1984; Stolorow, Atwood, & Brandchaft, 1987, 1994). My own contributions (Orange, Atwood, & Stolorow, 1997; Stolorow, Atwood, & Orange, 2002) began at about the time when Brandchaft started to pursue his work on systems of pathological accommodation more independently. Nevertheless, ties of friendship and of intersubjective clinical sensibility continue among all of us. I remain deeply grateful for the opportunity to work with these eminent thinkers and clinicians and for the support they have given me.

development and treatment as occurring in the intricate interface between the experiential worlds of the persons involved. Let us listen to one formulation of Brandchaft's (1991) version:

> Because the experience of each of the players (analyst and patient) is shaped not only by the circumstance the patient presents to the analyst but by the triggering effect on the analyst's ways of organizing his experience and the unconscious principles determining these modes, the analytic commitment to seek to understand the experience of patients from a perspective within the patient's subjective framework acquires a new and expanded meaning. Failures of the analyst from within the patient's subjective experience, the particular meanings encoded in that experience, what is revived and precisely how it has come to be organized, will all ultimately have to occupy the focus of the kind of sustained self reflective inquiry [the therapist] initiated in himself. (p. 103)*

Before Brandchaft begins to consider the developmental story of intersubjectivity, so familiar to him from his studies with Kohut and Winnicott and his long discussions with Stolorow and Atwood, he always already begins from the clinical situation. First he sees the face of a devastated human being, and next, equipped with an intersubjective developmental sensibility, so congenial to a hermeneutics of trust, he begins to wonder how this happened. At every moment, he tells us, we must first and last attend to our impact on the patient and refrain from blaming the patient for whatever the patient says or does. (Dostoyevsky and Lévinas: I am always responsible!) Brandchaft knows that his involvement never suspends long enough for him to diagnose or pathologize "the patient." The continuous and intricate mutuality of the clinical situation finds its exact parallel in early development:

---

* For readers unfamiliar with intersubjective systems theory's clinical practice, see Stolorow et al. (1987). For the philosophical underpinnings, see Atwood and Stolorow (1984) and Stolorow and Atwood (1992). For a very short and easy introduction, see the first chapter of Orange et al. (1997).

The unconscious principles that organize experience and give it its distinctive stamp ... begin to be established very early in life, some time before the capacity for symbolic thought has been achieved. They are determined by the specific conditions or rules that the child experiences as governing his role in the mutual regulation of affectively harmonious relationships with his important caretakers. Breaking these rules and violating these conditions involves renunciation of the only source of comfort within the child's experience. These unconscious principles thereupon provide an unequalled opportunity and otherwise unavailable window into most basic and affect laden childhood experiences, the residues of these, and the impact upon the child's developmental architecture. (1991, pp. 103–104)

The hermeneutics of trust might seem deceptively easier than the hermeneutics of suspicion with all its elaborate decoding, but not so. The hermeneutics of trust requires us to watch and listen carefully for these signs of our impact on the so-called opposition of the patient, whose depressive response to our subtle coercion or pulls for compliance needs to be read as the heroic resistance we discussed previously. In its place, in Brandchaft's (1993) own words,

> it becomes mandatory that the analytic process reinstate the developmental process at the point at which it was interrupted. This necessarily involves the analysis providing a setting in which the patient can live through whatever anxiety lies in the path of his reclaiming the ownership of his self and determining the laws by which his sense and definition of self are governed. Only in that way will it be possible for him at last to depend upon another without placing himself at risk of surrendering the determination of who he is to that other. (p. 226)

This process will inevitably involve sincere self-scrutiny on the analyst's part, even if it never amounts to a Ferenczian mutual analysis. Our personal and professional self-cohesion may depend, in a somewhat parental way, on trying to see the road ahead of our patients. In addition, we are full of values and biases that can never be fully absent from—indeed they often positively inform—our analytic work. Yet the hermeneutics of trust means learning from our patients how to set them free from us so that they may truly travel their own path.

Brandchaft has long noted that obsessional patients manifest the compulsive accommodation he describes in its purest and most tortured form. My patient Luke, for example, for several years showed just the deflated response that Brandchaft describes whenever I became impatient and interrupted his careful narratives and explanations, thinking we might be able to get to the point in fewer than the 40 minutes before I would be allowed to enter the conversation. Where some contemporary points of view might see Luke as attempting to control me, and recommend that I insist on being acknowledged, Brandchaft has taught me to understand him as heroically defending his very being against my impingement. Only when I was able to communicate to him the full and profound necessity for such defense, in the context of his developmental trauma, has it begun to soften. I am glad to report that our style of conversation has become much more dialogical in recent times.

THE HERMENEUTICS OF PATHOLOGICAL ACCOMMODATION

For many years many admiring students of Brandchaft agreed that we hated his expression "pathological accommodation" for his central idea. We knew that we all adjusted to others—sometimes more than we should, granted—and we did not want to be pathologized for it. Now, understanding his distinction from the ordinary and necessary* accommodating that forms part of everyday learning and relating, I am no longer among them. What he intends to describe for us truly deserves the name of illness and

---

* Shelley Doctors (2010), for example, explained that pathological accommodation results from relational trauma, whereas "to learn to adjust one's understandings and behavior to the context in which one lives is a normal part of life. A great deal of social/cultural learning takes place in this manner" (p. 5).

needs all our curative and healing effort or, in the more political terms that he and Stolorow have chosen, emancipatory effort.

Briefly, for those unfamiliar with Brandchaft's work, *pathological accommodation* means that, at the deepest levels of our being, we may have been co-opted into a choice between the bond we need or needed to the parent or parental system and our own personal existence. We then live, or half-live, reactively but not creatively, caged in patterns of rebellion or compliance, "imprisoned in gulags of [our] minds" (Brandchaft, 1993, p. 212). In his carefully chosen words, first presented in New York in 1991 to many of us who remember this occasion well,

> "Pre-emptory adhesion" to the dictates of caretakers gets internalized in a set of pathological accommodative principles that continue to operate automatically outside awareness to maintain archaic bonds. That is the route by which so many individuals in our culture have become isolated from an innermost essence of their own. Their subjective world is substantially constituted by a reality originally imposed from without. Awareness of inner experience does not occupy, and is not allowed to occupy, a central role in defining and consolidating the sense of self and in generating behavior. Alien constructs define and appraise the self, their origins buried in antiquity and impervious to new information. What emerges is an automatic, invariant, unexamined and unquestioned patterning which constitutes a major impediment to learning from experience and source of resistance to change in analysis. (Brandchaft, 2002, p. 729)

Unfortunately our psychoanalytic institutions, Brandchaft believes, almost always requiring profound self-abnegation as the cost of belonging, exactly replicate the familial systems of pathological accommodation. To me it seems that the professional life stories of the five groundbreakers we have studied in this book illustrate his contention well. Each walked a fine line between belonging and exile, in the service of responding to what each one saw as the need to put suffering people before "adherence to the dictates of Antiquity." Each remained attached to psychoanalysis, in other words to "antiquity" (Gadamer's "tradition," perhaps), without adhering or submitting to all of its "dictates" when the face of the suffering other called them out.

As we noted previously, Brandchaft has struggled lifelong for his own emancipation from one "dictate of antiquity" after another. It seems to me notable that an aspect of his interest in Winnicott concerned his (Winnicott's) efforts to free himself from the influence of Klein. Brandchaft's (1986) similar hermeneutic sensibility emerged when he wrote,

> Of his work with Melanie Klein, Winnicott recounts that he consulted her on the one analysis he had done on the basis of his own Strachey analysis and "went on to try to learn some of the immense amount she knew already. ... This was difficult for me," he wrote "because overnight I changed from being a pioneer [in pediatric psychiatry] into being a student with a pioneer teacher" (Winnicott, 1965, p. 173). Within the context of those times, it is easy to understand how he gradually came to focus increasingly on the contribution of environmental factors in development, when all around him the focus was so heavily on the biological and innate. His contributions reflect his personal attempt to return to his pioneering course and to free himself from some of the influences that undoubtedly governed his personal analysis with Riviere and his supervision in training under the formidable influence of Klein. His declarations that "there is no such thing as a baby" and that "infant and mother together form an indivisible unit" (Winnicott, 1965, p. 39) were the most emphatic challenges to the edifice Klein had built that an unshackled mind could proclaim. (p. 269)

We hear again the Brandchaft who can see the face and hear the voice of the imprisoned—especially in a theory as formidable as the Tower of London that one could imagine incarcerating those compelled to believe in it as the price of psychoanalytic belonging—but who can also notice and celebrate the emergence from prison of an "unshackled mind":

> The unique and brilliant contributions that marked the last years of [Winnicott's] life seem to me to reflect his own personal voyage from what was for him a false self to a more singular, unique, and creative true self. They signaled the end of a journey he well might

have characterized as from selfless dependence via relative dependence to mature independence. He cast these personal experiences into a theoretical model in which these concepts were elaborated. As lasting as his contributions are likely to be, one cannot read his works without being aware that he was never quite able to separate himself fully from the earlier influences. ... It is fascinating to read in Winnicott's work in 1962 the discovery that decisively marked his departure from the influence of Klein. "I must refer to the fact," he writes, "that in many cases the analyst displaces environmental influences that are pathological, and we gain insight of the kind that enables us to know when we have become modern representatives of the parent figures of the patient's childhood and infancy, and when by contrast we are displacing such figures." (pp. 269–270)

This extensive narrative deserves careful attention for two reasons. First, Brandchaft had been present in London and seen at close hand the overwhelming influence of Melanie Klein, perhaps one of the two most powerful figures in the history of psychoanalysis. He had watched Winnicott's struggles to free himself—long before he developed the language of pathological accommodation—and saw, once again in England, what pressures the psychoanalytic establishment could bring to bear. He saw that Winnicott never became completely free, but he already recognized in him the insight that both Winnicott and Brandchaft—perhaps unknowingly—shared with Ferenczi, that the analyst inevitably at times participates in the retraumatization of the patient. We displace the traumatizers and offer something healing, but we also, in the very next moment, repeat the original problematic situation. Winnicott found the courage, in 1962, to stand up and say this to the British Society, and Brandchaft did not forget.

Second, an easy fusion would equate Brandchaft's systems of pathological accommodation with Winnicott's false self based on compliance, and self-chosen path with the true self. But Brandchaft has rarely even alluded to this connection, and we must ask why. Probably he did not want to be misunderstood, as Winnicott has often been, as describing a superficial social conformity. Systems of pathological accommodation concern a usurpation of one's being at a level so basic that nothing is more fundamental; a false self, as both Winnicott and Brandchaft have understood, represents an attempt to survive without any sense of being real and without having any sense of being oneself. Both understood that the devastated others they met in their work had never had the opportunity to come into their own being or pursue their own path. They expected, like rebellious Martin, to be crushed again at every moment, especially once they began to trust the analyst as a new attachment possibility. Here is another moment where Brandchaft acknowledges his clear kinship with Winnicott's concepts:

> Clearer recognition of false and true self-structuring, which oscillates almost instantaneously in treatment, together with the elucidation of the triggering contexts in which these shifts take place, provides a richer latticework for the recognition of, and for an effective approach to the treatment of, structures of pathological accommodation. (Brandchaft et al., 2010, p. 199)

There is, however, no simple or solitary exit from the prison of what Brandchaft has called pathological accommodation. Only with the help of another who seeks to understand the terms of the incarceration, and probably another who has known this prison from the inside, can it come unlocked. But the analyst too may become tangled up in the accommodative prison, not even recognizing that she or he may be keeping the patient inside. Brandchaft (2007) wrote,

> The repetitive sequencing of such states of mind takes the form of obsessive brooding and self-reproach from which patients cannot free themselves when they are alone. These states are frequently not clearly recognized as discrete states of mind and as reactive to psychologically complex triggering interactions. ... Terror has been unleashed in the subjective world ... terror requires immediate preventive or preemptive intervention. However, in analysis, it is imperative that these states are clearly identified, and the analyst's reflective power restored if he is to avoid becoming entangled in a reifying ruminative process or in action/interpretation designed to terminate the offending state. (p. 674)

In the earlier story of Luke, I was tempted to "terminate the offending state" by finishing his sentences. With another patient, I might be tempted too quickly to reassure, without thoroughly understanding that the shame being expressed protected an absolutely needed bond. It is crucial that I begin to notice the ways in which I pull for the patient's compliance; in Lévinasian terms, I am unwittingly reducing instead of responding and thus I repeat the earlier murder instead of accompanying the sufferer so that he or she may not die alone.

We now turn to Brandchaft's central idea, so often misunderstood as referring to behavioral compliance. Much like Ferenczi's identification with the aggressor (Ferenczi, 1988; Ferenczi & Dupont, 1988)—not at all like the behavioral imitation described by Anna Freud (1967)—Brandchaft's "pathological accommodation" describes a takeover* of the developing child's whole being:

> Within traumatic attachment systems ... the traumatized child has come to feel itself as bad. Its experience has been interlaced with threats and episodes of abandonment, physical and psychological, and first belief in causality establishes that it has done something egregiously, malignantly and selfishly "wrong." The child has been forced to adopt or embrace, this alien impinging referent as not-to-be-questioned Truth because such threats leave it helpless. Intense anxiety is roused, and the anger generated is the only means the child possesses to attempt to prevent the caregiver from carrying out or continuing the threat. Subsequently, when its anger is ignored or thrown back and the child blamed for the difficulty, a dysfunctional hermetic feedback circuitry has been firmly established. Chronic rage and revenge follow. ... The child carries the stigma of badness driven into his selfhood and will never be able to put the torment to rest: "Like damn little men pounding at my brain with picks and axes and chisels." (Brandchaft, 2007, pp. 674–675)

---

* Thomas Ogden (1982) provided a similar account of how this comes about, writing of "...the pressure on an infant to behave in a manner congruent with the mother's pathology, and the ever-present threat that if the infant fails to comply, he would cease to exist for the mother. This threat is the muscle behind the demand for compliance: 'If you are not what I need you to be, you don't exist for me.' Or in other language, 'I can see in you only what I put there. If I don't see that, I see nothing'" (p. 16).

Only a clinician equipped with the hermeneutics of trust could hear this torture behind the rage and vengefulness that one is tempted to disparage as "resistance." In Brandchaft's emancipatory psychoanalysis we come to recognize that a hermeneutics of trust leads to compassion for our suffering patients, for our candidates and younger colleagues who fear imprisonment by the "psychoanalytic police." We may even embrace his compassionate hermeneutics for ourselves as we, like Brandchaft, engage in our lifelong struggles to hear with our own ears, to see with our own eyes, to speak with our own voices what we are not allowed to hear, see, and speak. From him, we find courage to fight free from "the dictates of Antiquity," reminding ourselves that this is indeed the attitude of heroes.

FORMS OF PATHOLOGICAL ACCOMMODATION

The best way to get a feel for what Brandchaft means by pathological accommodation, of the range of its manifestations, and—worst of all—of its tenacity is to read his extended clinical accounts of the intractably depressed composer, of Patrick the hopeless architect, of Marco the melancholic playwright, and of Martin, who, if he had been 10 years old, would likely have received a diagnosis of oppositional defiant disorder.* Though my own favorite remains the depressed composer, Brandchaft's most compact description is of the successful architect Patrick, married, father of three children, who also appeared successful but was tormented by depression and a sense of complete futility. The first task of the hermeneutics of trust is often to recognize the suffering of people whose lives look enviable, even to therapists. Just as the poet Theodore Roethke wrote, "I would believe my pain," we learn to believe the misery and devastation of the other, even when it may

---

* Though Brandchaft wrote of men, Shelley Doctors added accounts of women to make it clear that the ideas apply easily across gender lines (Brandchaft et al., 2010).

be discounted by the world around and by the patient's family. Brandchaft (1993) asked,

> What was it that continued to agonize Patrick so cruelly? He was the eldest son of a father who had freed himself from his own childhood impoverishment to become a legend in the ranks of pioneer developers of housing tracts and shopping centers, a man who had amassed undreamed-of wealth. The father attempted to pass on the lessons life had taught him to his son, whom he loved, with the same tenacity that had served him so successfully in his business affairs. He espoused the virtues of hard work with a missionary ardor, and he heaped scorn and predictions of apocalypse upon anyone whose zeal in this direction was less than his own. Attention to detail he elevated to the status of the nuclear art form. "Make certain you do the little things," he would preach, "and the big things will follow." As a boy, Patrick had drawn the unfortunate "little thing" assignment of raking the leaves of their fine new house each afternoon after school. In the evening before the family could sit down to supper, dad would accompany the lad into the yard and inspect the results of his labors. No white-gloved marine sergeant was more dedicated to his task. His father's reproaches and his own forebodings as neglected leaves were discovered and pointed to, his indolence or fraudulence thus unmasked, remained indelibly seared in Patrick's memory. (p. 213)

Listening to Patrick, one can feel the darkness closing in. No space exists for spontaneity, for enjoyment, for a self-chosen task. The question always hovers and impends: Has it been done perfectly? Only if so can the tenuous bond to the other be maintained until the next mistake.

> Patrick's father could not understand why he should be having such difficulties in getting his firstborn son to follow simple instructions. Equally difficult for him to comprehend was how Patrick could find appealing any interests or entertain any ambitions other than those he had determined were in the boy's best interest. ... He especially could not understand why the boy was so offended whenever they visited one of his new development projects. ... Patrick could only see mindless and garish desecration being inflicted on the environment, and having experienced it at shorter range on himself, he reacted viscerally. Although dad

regularly and cordially invited Patrick to come along on his fishing trips or sailing boat excursions, he never attended a baseball game in which his son, who took pride in his feats as a second baseman, was playing. (p. 213)

It is tempting to study the structure of Brandchaft's elegant narrative; instead let us simply notice that he has allowed himself to be drawn into understanding his patient's predicament. One can already sense the deflated 10-year-old and what a lonely* "gulag" his life is becoming:

> This schism between what he saw and felt and what he was supposed to see and feel ... created an architecture for his spirit that was almost as confining as his life with father had ever been. Patrick could never really unlearn very much of what his father had insisted on teaching him. Any spontaneous enthusiasm or fun for anything he might design for himself, including his own lifestyle, came inexorably to be erased, automatically and mysteriously, as if by some unseen master hand and as if it—and, in a profound sense, he—had never really existed. (p. 214)

We said earlier that pathological accommodation bears almost no resemblance to ordinary social conformity—speaking one's own language, driving on the customary side of the street, and so on. Instead, for the sake of survival† it erases—by an act of murder, Lévinas or Shengold might say—the child who would otherwise be coming into his own. Ferenczi might have recognized in systems of pathological accommodation the confusion of tongues stabilized and automatized. As Patrick lived in his profession,

---

* Stephen Mitchell (1986) once described a process much like Brandchaft's pathological accommodation but attributed it to the costs of idealizing: "Although this is an oversimplified account of religion [Feuerbach's], idealization in human relations often does reflect this masochistic, projective process. Because of disturbed earlier relationships, there is a terror of individuation and self-development. The analysand fears that finding his own path means isolation, a feature often originating in the context of relationships with parents who demand adoration and deference as the price of involvement. For such an analysand, the only way to insure human contact is to find someone to go first, to remain always in someone's shadow" (pp. 129–130).
† Brandchaft, without much interest in attachment categories, takes completely seriously Bowlby's view that humans need attachment for survival. We will thus accept terrible conditions to keep needed bonds.

there was no time and no space for the enjoyment of his superbly innovative spirit. He had to concern himself with every detail of any project he undertook, as if it were the lawn that was to be inspected by his father. Patrick drew each design and bird-dogged it through the detailed drafting process. He took the plans to the building authorities himself and personally followed the interminable procedures necessary to secure the required permits. He even had to see that the garbage was taken to the street from his office himself, for he was certain that anyone to whom he delegated the responsibility would forget it sooner or later. If he departed in the slightest from this ritualized existence, he was filled with terrible foreboding. He was compelled to conclude what his father had always maintained—that his insistence on choosing his own life for himself and not accepting what his father chose for him was an unarguable demonstration of his stupidity or willfulness. (p. 214)

The phenomenological description of this "gulag" leads easily to its interpretation within Brandchaft's particular version of a hermeneutics of trust. In other words, we see the patient's obsessional thinking and compulsive behavior as a desperate attempt to survive his psychological confinement in an isolation cell where perfection buys him only an extended sentence, but nothing that could be called more than "life imprisonment." Most important, Patrick showed his analyst how this whole system of pathological accommodation worked so that they could begin to understand and very slowly modify it together:

What happened in my consulting room, I was able to determine, was a faithful replication of what occurred when Patrick was by himself. Observing how his mental operations always came to ground zero in this repetitive self-negating process, I got a vivid sense of how like a cell Patrick's mind was. I could observe how each time the cell door opened with a fresh, innovative thought or exuberant feeling it soon clanged shut again. Only by immersing himself in work to the point of exhaustion had Patrick been able to find some measure of relief from this process. (pp. 214–215)

Other patients, like Martin who always arrived late, showed an oppositional form of this original self-destruction. Much like those Kohut had understood in his descriptions of narcissistic rage, when the sense of self was so endangered, only antagonistic insistence could keep them feeling that they existed at all.

Some patients alternated between Martin's defiant belligerence and the sad deflation we see in Patrick and in the composer of "intractable depression," both forms of the resistance that Brandchaft, in a *tour de force* of the hermeneutics of trust, calls "the attitude of heroes." There is nothing obviously heroic in antagonism or passivity, but Brandchaft can see the refusal of a life conceded to the demands of a Faustian bargain. In the alternators, at both ends of the pendulum swing, Brandchaft perceives the courageous effort to survive psychologically. In his own words,

> I have come to recognize this constellation of shifting feeling states as an indication that there is an underlying process at work—ghosts, as it were—that discloses skeletons below ... one of the two sets of perspectives and motivations, that which divests the self of what is exquisitely personal, is always preprogrammed to prevail. Thus, development on the basis of authenticity of experience and centrality of differentiated choice is repetitively foreclosed. (p. 215)

In these shifting constellations, we can recognize not only psychiatric "bipolarity" but also familiar alternations between frustrated defiance and deflated despair, in everyday clinical experience, and perhaps in our own lives.

RETHINKING OBSESSIONALITY FROM THE HERMENEUTICS OF TRUST

Brandchaft's generous hermeneutic revolutionizes our understanding of obsessionality by placing it within what I have called in previous chapters a hermeneutic of trauma:

> In cases of severe developmental trauma we are dealing with a qualitatively different organization of experience from that for which the prolonged focus on intrapsychic neurotic conflict [between instinctual impulses and superego prohibitions] had prepared us. In agreement with attachment theorists, I have come to believe that such trauma constitutes an assault on nuclear formations of the personality from the outset. ... Trauma acts relentlessly to undermine the construction of the context of security that is indispensable to the child if it is to develop a nuclear sense of confidence and purposefulness in its own being and expression. (Brandchaft, 2002, p. 734)

The infant, child, or adult in a traumatized state, if not stunned and frozen, scans the environment ceaselessly, looking for indications of further danger. This means, in our common clinical experience, that patients ask us the same question over and over again, like babies who cannot be comforted. They cannot be comforted, because, as Brandchaft pointed out, trauma has assaulted the basic context of security that would make any answer to a question, or any reassurance to the terrified child, usable for self-soothing and for building up a sense of self and direction. Instead we have obsessionality, the terror of making decisions that could be wrong and have disastrous consequences. The obsessionally inclined person fears doing something to trigger the original traumatic situation and tries compulsively to do everything right to prevent a recurrence. The child, and later the adult, becomes painfully sensitized to the possible disapproval of others, especially of those who "matter." "When the threat of trauma becomes preoccupying for the child, the maintenance of the attachment becomes compelling, and processes of pathological accommodation may become organized" (Brandchaft et al., 2010, p. 170), "to keep maladjustment in good repair" (p. 171). At best, one lives very carefully. Ordinary development of one's own purposes and projects, in the context of good-enough attachment security, becomes impossible or at least deferred for some future time when it might become safer. Of course this time never comes. Instead, Brandchaft (2002) tells us,

> A proto sensitivity to triggering cues will have been built in because the child's ability to depend on caregiver protection has been seriously undermined by the primitive context in which caregivers and traumatizers were one. The child will therefore come selectively to include and exclude such cues. ... No substantive change can take place so long as these primary defense systems remain intact in unrecognized, split off or dissociated forms. *It is mandatory, therefore, that a relational bond of security be established as the primary goal and essential foundation for continuing therapeutic interaction and transformation.* (p. 735, emphasis in original)

This risk avoidance can range from an attunement and adjustment that shuts down one's own creativity to the kinds of obsessions and compulsions that build seriously locked-down prisons. A sufferer

> continues selectively to cling to noxious external relational ties and experience self-endangerment when these come under threat. In the inner world, similarly exhausting obsessive ruminations cannot be relinquished because they carry the unrecognized proxies for the insecure attachments of childhood. Obsessional preoccupations become "state-entrapment systems" because the person is unable to recognize them as trauma-produced disregulative disorders of the thinking process itself, just as he was unable to recognize the patterns of traumatic impingement, neglect and abuse as rooted in disregulated thought disorders of his caregivers. He continues to feel them as oracular prognostications and they serve automatically to initiate coercive organizations of thought and ritualized behavior. (Brandchaft, 2001, p. 263)

In other words, the trauma is written everywhere, foreclosing every exit, making every moment of relaxing into simple enjoyment impossible. Everywhere there will be judgment, humiliation, devastation, loss beyond the possibility to sustain, unspeakable trauma. Worst of all, these dire "prognostications" all hang on desperately needed attachments.

In my experience as clinician and supervisor, seriously obsessional patients test our clinical patience and generous intentions. They go on and on, worrying about the same questions for days and weeks and years. Often with them we lack the experience of being engaged in dialogue, and our warm and welcoming hermeneutics of trust goes right out the window. So let us listen to the way that Brandchaft (2001) hears their traumatized voices:

> In obsessional disorders, a relentless underlying self-hatred exists, even when it is disguised beneath compulsive cravings for constant reassurances of love and affirmation. ... However, beneath such self-hatred are to be found profound feelings of worthlessness and despair at one's utter failure to have brought joy into the lives of caregivers, when nothing else has been found to give meaning to existence, theirs and one's own. (pp. 265–266)

Brandchaft's hermeneutic ear hears the compulsive symptom as self-hatred for failure at tasks that should never have belonged to a child. (In families where terrible retribution could follow the stealing of eighteen cents, the loss of small amounts of grocery money, the reaching for food, or the wrong haircut, children grow up to live in secret terror that never ends.) Once again, we see that systems of pathological accommodation memorialize—and in obsessions and compulsions, freeze in place—what Ferenczi called the confusion of tongues. (I suspect that these patients somehow did not manage the escape that Ferenczi described in his "wise baby" dreams—see Chapter 3—but rather remained frozen in a traumatic either–or.) Brandchaft continued,

> *Primal failure* and *incurable defect* have been transgenerationally transmitted from within an incompetent developmental system, to become installed at the very core of the child's "being." They cannot be let go of, for somehow they have become both the defining link and protective talisman. When the child attempts to throw off shackles of abuse or accommodation, enveloping and spiraling obsessional ruminative states appear. The loss of object [attachment figure] foreshadows terrifying states of estrangement and encroaching non-existence. *Even rebellion or protective withdrawal are accompanied by a sense of worthlessness so that traumatizer and traumatized remain as one.* (p. 266, emphasis added)

Brandchaft here makes sense, through trusting the obsessional patient's symptoms to make sense and not to reflect resistance to the analysis, of several disparate clinical phenomena. First, the shame and self-hatred often emerges as a terror of making mistakes, as if mistakes and failure would be tragic. Indeed they are in a system of relational trauma structured into a should–should not system in which any mistake means the last hope of personal survival may be lost. One may be excluded from the human world entirely. No wonder one must stand paralyzed if too many choices face one.

Second, the threat of loss—for any reason—means life and death. When bonds are so tenuous in the beginning, and so dependent on the erasure of the child, then every possibility of loss looms like death. Most of my suicidally obsessional patients had early parental loss added to the developmental trauma of which Brandchaft tells, and they have been almost exactly describable in the terms he uses. Often anorexics, dangerously ill, have been terrified of dying from one misstep, but they are unsure what would constitute that misstep. The immediate focus on food and weight often obscures the underlying sources of the terror. Only by understanding the original relational traumatic system, as well as the compounding of the incomprehensible losses, have we been able to pull them back from the brink.

Third, Brandchaft notes that these patients often blame themselves for not having been able to bring joy into the lives of their caregivers and, by extension in my experience, for not having been able to keep the caregiver alive—emotionally, physically, or both. They therefore often bear a profound sense that they deserve to die themselves and are scanning for news of their own impending demise. Even if they live, they have never done their "duty" and are never permitted to "go on being," to let the world be their oyster, even for five minutes.

Fourth, at the heart of the child's being—and Brandchaft, like the others, knows that he and his patients are both children and adults—live, in full installations, *primal failure* and *incurable defect*. Frieda Fromm-Reichmann used to say, only half in jest, that in Germany, one says, "I have failure," whereas in America, one says, "I am a failure" and that she could not imagine why anyone here would ever attempt anything. Brandchaft refers to this sense, more or less profound and pervasive, that one *is* a failure at the core of one's being, because one has failed one's parents, usually from long before one could imagine what that means. He therefore taught us to notice carefully the signs of emotional deflation—so well-known to the infant researchers—that occur in our work when our response or lack of response retraumatizes our patient.

THE TRUST THAT LIBERATES

This leads, finally, to the treatment implications of Brandchaft's account of obsessionality in particular and of pathological accommodation in general. In treatment, one begins to try to "throw off the shackles," and then the demons really come out. As Brandchaft and many of us have noticed, "enveloping and spiraling obsessional ruminative states appear," and patients often feel that treatment is making them worse (see Brandchaft, 1983, on the so-called negative therapeutic reaction). It requires a clinician alert to the precise dangers—of relational retraumatization—that Brandchaft describes to meet and hold (in the Winnicottian sense) the patient in these moments of terror. If the patient accuses me of injuring him or her, or simply regards me with fear, it is up to me to stay engaged. Moreover, Brandchaft insists, I must ask myself what I am doing or not doing, saying or not saying, to terrify the patient. We are intertwined together in this prison, and only together can we find a way out.

Again, however, we easily become impatient, setting off the patient's terror. Even acknowledging progress can mean to the patient that, after all, loss and abandonment are just around the corner. Allowing oneself to feel somewhat secure, and to begin to seek one's own path, turned out to be the same old trap after all. So we find such declarations of progress often create clinical havoc:

> I have emphasized the tenacity of the "resistance to change" that accompanies a liberating fundamental shift. The resistance appears in the form of an intolerable anxiety, finding expression in a variety of channels, whenever the patient enters the domain of specific transformational change. Growing feelings of estrangement and loss embedded in the departure from the matrix of developmental attachments signaled by the opening of new pathways of experience may combine with increased fears of abandonment by, or loss of, the analyst to create an anticipation of unbearable pain and inconsolable grief. Fundamental change involves departures from life-long habituation to familiar sequences and modes of feeling, thinking and being. … Advances in the patient's understanding regularly appear to vanish when he once more comes under the grip of an obsessive danger. (Brandchaft, 2001, p. 284)

So we regroup, without shaming or blaming the patient, and realize that our desire to succeed, to be helpful, to feel some satisfaction in our work has terrified our vulnerable, loss-ravaged patient. In the unassuming spirit characteristic of Brandchaft's response to the face of the suffering stranger, we proceed more gently:

> When one is able to become reasonably comfortable in continuing to wonder and pursue the investigation of what is happening, in the place of discomfort in comparisons with what "should be" and is not taking place, change will frequently emerge. Evidence of such change is for the most part silent, slow, precarious and incremental, and it is more likely to occur when it "just happens" and is not being looked for. It may also sometimes turn out to be not the basis for retreat but for more enduring and far-reaching growth. (pp. 284–285)

Brandchaft expressed simply and elegantly here the hermeneutics of trust. Another example, from the correspondence of Hannah Arendt with her husband, Heinrich Blücher, takes on special poignancy in the context of her complex and apparently much less liberating relationship with Martin Heidegger (Maier-Katkin, 2010). She wrote to Blücher,

I can only truly exist in love. And that is why I was so frightened that I might simply get lost. And so I made myself independent. And about the love of others who branded me as coldhearted, I always thought: if you only knew how dangerous love would be for me. Then when I met you, suddenly I was no longer afraid. … It still seems incredible to me that I managed to get both things, the "love of my life" and a oneness with myself. And yet, I only got one thing when I got the other. But finally I also know what happiness is. (p. 109)

Afterword: The Next Step

The implications of this book's thesis, that dialogic understanding, in a hermeneutic of trust, forms the hospitable response to the suffering stranger demanded by the ethics of infinite responsibility, clearly extend beyond our "everyday clinical practice" into the larger worlds where suffering and injustice collide every day. In addition, these contexts of injustice and cruelty shape our "everyday clinical practice" and the assumptions we bring to it. Fortunately, other clinicians and theorists more grounded than I in political theory, in social ethics, and in cross-cultural/religious understanding are already courageously exploring these challenges.

Meanwhile, in my view, Buber was right: To redeem one person *is* to redeem the world or at least to make a beginning. To provide a warm, hospitable, and dialogic welcome for the frozen, stunned, and nearly dead is a quiet and unspectacular task. To respond to the face of *this* suffering sister or brother is my ethical work, good clinical practice, the work of understanding that gives the other the benefit of the doubt. *Hineni.*

References

Alford, C. (2007). Lévinas, Winnicott, and therapy. *Psychoanalytic Review, 94,* 529–551.

Altman, N. (1998). Book review: Freely associated: Encounters in psychoanalysis with Christopher Bollas, Joyce McDougall, Michael Eigen, Adam Phillips, and Nina Coltart. Edited by Anthony Molino. New York: Free Association Books 1997 (211 pp.). *Psychoanalytic Review, 85,* 943–947.

Apel, K.-O. (1971). *Hermeneutik und Ideologiekritik.* Frankfurt am Main: Suhrkamp.

Aristotle, B. S., & Davis, M. (2002). *Aristotle on poetics.* South Bend, IN: St. Augustine's Press.

Aron, L. (1992). From Ferenczi to Searles and contemporary relational approaches: Commentary on Mark Blechner's "Working in the countertransference." *Psychoanalytic Dialogues, 2*(2), 181–190.

Aron, L., & Frankel, J. (1994). Who is overlooking whose reality? Commentary on Tabin's "Freud's shift from the seduction theory: Some overlooked reality factors." *Psychoanalytic Psychology, 11*(2), 291–302.

Aron, L., & Harris, A. (1993). *The legacy of Sándor Ferenczi.* Hillsdale, NJ: Analytic Press.

Atterton, P., Calarco, M., & Friedman, M. S. (2004). *Lévinas and Buber: Dialogue and difference.* Pittsburgh, PA: Duquesne University Press.

Atwood, G. (2010). The abyss of madness: An interview. *International Journal of Psychoanalytic Self Psychology, 5,* 334–356.

Atwood, G. E., & Stolorow, R. D. (1984). *Structures of subjectivity: Explorations in psychoanalytic phenomenology.* Hillsdale, NJ: Analytic Press.

Atwood, G. E., & Stolorow, R. D. (1993). *Faces in a cloud: Intersubjectivity in personality theory.* Northvale, NJ: Jason Aronson.

Bacciagaluppi, M. (1994). The influence of Ferenczi on Bowlby. *International Forum of Psychoanalysis, 3*(2), 97–101.

Baker, H., & Jones, S. (2008). Adding a spiritual dimension to the biopsychosocial model: Psychoanalysis, Heinz Kohut, Friedrich Schleiermacher, Martin Buber and Gabriel Marcel. *Transdisciplinarity in Science and Religion, 4,* 135–171.

Balint, M. (1957a). *Problems of human pleasure and behaviour.* New York: Liveright.

Balint, M. (1957b). *Problems of human pleasure and behaviour.* London: Hogarth Press.

Balint, M. (1958). Sándor Ferenczi's last years. *The International Journal of Psychoanalysis, 39,* 68.

Balint, M. (1968). *The basic fault: Therapeutic aspects of regression.* London: Tavistock.

Bass, A. (2001). It takes one to know one: Or, whose unconscious is it anyway? *Psychoanalytic Dialogues, 11*(5), 683–702.

Beebe, B. (2000). Coconstructing mother–infant distress. *Psychoanalytic Inquiry, 20*(3), 421–440.

Beebe, B., & Lachmann, F. M. (1988). The contribution of mother–infant mutual influence to the origins of self- and object representations. *Psychoanalytic Psychology, 5*(4), 305–337.

Beebe, B., & Lachmann, F. M. (2001). *Infant research and adult treatment: A dyadic systems approach.* Hillsdale, NJ: Analytic Press.

Benjamin, J. (2000). Intersubjective distinctions: Subjects and persons, recognitions and breakdowns. *Psychoanalytic Dialogues, 10*(1), 43–55.

Benjamin, J. (2010). Can we recognize each other? Response to Donna Orange. *International Journal of Psychoanalytic Self Psychology, 5,* 244–256.

Berman, E. (2002). Identifying with the other: A conflictual, vital necessity. *Psychoanalytic Dialogues, 12*(1), 141–151.

Berman, E. (2004). Sándor, Gizella, Elma: A biographical journey. *The International Journal of Psychoanalysis, 85,* 489–520.

Bernanos, G., & Morris, P. (1937). *The diary of a country priest.* New York: Macmillan.

Bernasconi, R., & Wood, D. (1988). *The provocation of Lévinas: Rethinking the other.* New York: Routledge.

Bókay, A. (1998). Turn of fortune in psychoanalysis. *International Forum of Psychoanalysis, 7*(4), 189–199.
Bollas, C. (1989). *Forces of destiny: Psychoanalysis and human idiom*. London: Free Association Books.
Bonhoeffer, D. (1995). *The cost of discipleship*. New York: Touchstone.
Bonomi, C. (1998). Jones's allegation of Ferenczi's mental deterioration. *International Forum of Psychoanalysis, 7*(4), 201–206.
Bonomi, C. (1999). Flight into sanity. *International Journal of Psychoanalysis, 80*(3), 507–542.
Bonomi, C. (2002). Identification with the aggressor: An interactive tactic or an intrapsychic tomb? *Psychoanalytic Dialogues, 12*(1), 153–158.
Borgogno, F. (2004). Why Ferenczi today? The contribution of Sándor Ferenczi to the understanding and healing of psychic suffering. *International Forum of Psychoanalysis, 13*, 5–13.
Boulanger, G. (2002). The cost of survival. *Contemporary Psychoanalysis, 38*(1), 17–44.
Bowie, A. (2002, July/August). Obituary: Hans-Georg Gadamer, 1900–2002. *Radical Philosophy*. Retrieved from http://www.radicalphilosophy.com/default.asp?channel_id=2191&editorial_id=10615
Bowlby, J. (1979). *The making and breaking of affectional bonds*. London: Tavistock.
Brabant, E., Falzeder, E., & Giampieri-Deutsch, P. (1993). *The correspondence of Sigmund Freud and Sándor Ferenczi Volume 1, 1908–1914*. Cambridge, MA: Harvard University Press.
Brandchaft, B. (1983). The negativism of the negative therapeutic reaction and the psychology of the self. In A. Goldberg (Ed.), *The future of psychoanalysis* (pp. 327–359). New York: International Universities Press.
Brandchaft, B. (1985). Discussion. *Progress in Self Psychology, 1*, 88–96.
Brandchaft, B. (1986). British object relations theory and self psychology. *Progress in Self Psychology, 2*, 245–272.
Brandchaft, B. (1988). A case of intractable depression. *Progress in Self Psychology, 4*, 133–154.
Brandchaft, B. (1991). Countertransference in the analytic process. *Progress in Self Psychology, 7*, 99–105.
Brandchaft, B. (1993). To free the spirit from its cell. *Progress in Self Psychology, 9*, 209–230.
Brandchaft, B. (2001). Obsessional disorders. *Psychoanalytic Inquiry, 21*(2), 253–288.
Brandchaft, B. (2002). Reflections on the intersubjective foundations of the sense of self. *Psychoanalytic Dialogues, 12*(5), 727–745.

Brandchaft, B. (2007). Systems of pathological accommodation and change in analysis. *Psychoanalytic Psychology, 24,* 667–687.

Brandchaft, B., Doctors, S., & Sorter, D. (2010). *Toward an emancipatory psychoanalysis: Brandchaft's intersubjective vision.* New York: Routledge.

Bromberg, P. (2006). *Awakening the dreamer: Clinical journeys.* Hillsdale, NJ: The Analytic Press.

Buber, M., & Buber Agassi, J. (1999). *Martin Buber on psychology and psychotherapy: Essays, letters, and dialogue.* New York: Syracuse University Press.

Bubner, R. (1994). On the ground of understanding. In B. Wachterhauser (Ed.), *Hermeneutics and truth* (pp. 68–82). Evanston, IL: Northwestern University Press.

Buechler, S. (1998). The analyst's experience of loneliness. *Contemporary Psychoanalysis, 34*(1), 91–113.

Buechler, S. (2009). Love will do the thing that's right: Commentary on paper by Stuart A. Pizer. *Psychoanalytic Dialogues, 19,* 63–68.

Buechler, S. (2010). No pain, no gain? Suffering and the analysis of defense. *Contemporary Psychoanalysis, 46,* 334–354.

Cassell, E. J. (2004). *The nature of suffering and the goals of medicine* (2nd ed.). New York: Oxford University Press.

Celenza, A. (1998). Precursors to therapist sexual misconduct. *Psychoanalytic Psychology, 15*(3), 378–395.

Celenza, A. (2010). The analyst's need and desire. *Psychoanalytic Dialogues, 20,* 60–69.

Chalier, C. (2002). *What ought I to do? Morality in Kant and Lévinas.* Ithaca, NY: Cornell University Press.

Chanter, T. (2001). *Feminist interpretations of Emmanuel Lévinas.* University Park: Pennsylvania State University Press.

Coburn, W. J. (2002). A world of systems. *Psychoanalytic Inquiry, 22*(5), 655–677.

Cohen, R. A. (1986). *Face to face with Lévinas.* Albany: State University of New York Press.

Courtois, C. A., & Ford, J. D. (2009). *Treating complex traumatic stress disorders: An evidence-based guide.* New York: Guilford.

Critchley, S. (2007). *Infinitely demanding: Ethics of commitment, politics of resistance.* London: Verso.

Critchley, S. (2002). Introduction. In S. Critchley & R. Bernasconi (Eds.), *The Cambridge Companion to Lévinas* (pp. 1–32). Cambridge, UK: Cambridge University Press.

Davey, N. (2006). *Unquiet understanding: Gadamer's philosophical hermeneutics.* Albany: State University of New York Press.

Davidson, D. (1984). *Inquiries into truth and interpretation.* New York: Oxford University Press.

Derrida, J. (1978). *Writing and difference.* Chicago: University of Chicago Press.

Dilthey, W., Makkreel, R. A., & Rodi, F. (2002). *The formation of the historical world in the human sciences.* Princeton, NJ: Princeton University Press.

Doctors, S. (2010, October). *An introduction of* Toward an emancipatory psychoanalysis: Brandchaft's intersubjective vision. Paper presented at the International Conference on the Psychology of the Self, Antalya, Turkey.

Donne, John. (1839) Meditation 17 in Henry Alford (Ed.), *The Works of John Donne* (pp. 574–575).Vol III. London: John W. Parker.

Dostal, R. (1987). The world never lost: The hermeneutics of trust. *Philosophy and Phenomenological Research, 47,* 413–434.

Dostal, R. (1994). The experience of truth for Gadamer and Heidegger: Taking time and sudden lightening. In B. Wachterhauser (Ed.), *Hermeneutics and truth* (pp. 47–67). Evanston, IL: Northwestern University Press.

Dostal, R. (Ed.). (2002). *The Cambridge companion to Gadamer.* Cambridge, UK: Cambridge University Press.

Dupont, I. (1988). Ferenczi's "madness." *Contemporary Psychoanalysis, 24,* 250–261.

Dupont, J. (1994). Freud's analysis of Ferenczi as revealed by their correspondence. *International Journal of Psychoanalysis, 75,* 301–320.

Dupont, J. (1998). The concept of trauma according to Ferenczi and its effects on subsequent psychoanalytical research. *International Forum of Psychoanalysis, 7*(4), 235–240.

Ellis, M., & O'Connor, N. (2010). *Questioning identities: Philosophy in psychoanalytic practice.* London: Karnac.

Erwin, E. (2002). *The Freud encyclopedia: Theory, therapy, and culture.* New York: Routledge.

Falzeder, E., & Brabant, E. (2000). *The correspondence of Sigmund Freud and Sándor Ferenczi, Volume 3, 1920–1933.* Cambridge, MA: Harvard University Press.

Falzeder, E., Brabant, E., & Giampieri-Deutsch, P. (1996). *The correspondence of Sigmund Freud and Sándor Ferenczi, Volume 2, 1914–1919.* Cambridge, MA: Harvard University Press.

Ferenczi, S. (1929). The unwelcome child and his death-instinct. *International Journal of Psychoanalysis, 10,* 125–129.

Ferenczi, S. (1930). The principle of relaxation and neocatharsis. *International Journal of Psychoanalysis, 11*, 428–443.

Ferenczi, S. (1931). Child-analysis in the analysis of adults. *International Journal of Psychoanalysis, 12*, 468–482.

Ferenczi, S. (1949a). Confusion of the tongues between the adults and the child (The language of tenderness and of passion). *International Journal of Psychoanalysis, 30*, 225–230.

Ferenczi, S. (1949b). Notes and fragments (1930–32). *International Journal of Psychoanalysis, 30*, 231–242.

Ferenczi, S. (1980). *Further contributions to the theory and technique of psycho-analysis.* New York: Brunner/Mazel.

Ferenczi, S., & Dupont, J. (1988). *The clinical diary of Sándor Ferenczi.* Cambridge, MA: Harvard University Press.

Ferenczi, S., Fortune, C., & Groddeck, G. (2001). *The Ferenczi–Georg Groddeck correspondence, 1921–1933.* New York: Other Press.

Fortune, C. (1993). The case of "RN": Sándor Ferenczi's radical experiment in psychoanalysis. In L. Aron & A. Harris (Eds.), *The legacy of Sándor Ferenczi* (pp. 101–120). Hillsdale, NJ: Analytic Press.

Frank, M. (1977). *Das individuelle Allgemeine: Textstrukturierung u. -interpretation nach Schleiermacher* (1. Aufl. ed.). Frankfurt am Main: Suhrkamp.

Frank, M. (1999). Style in philosophy, Part I. *Metaphilosophy, 30*, 145–167.

Frank, M. (2000). Self-awareness and self-knowledge: Mental familiarity and epistemic self-ascription. In W. Van Reijen & W. G. Weststeijn (Eds.), *Subjectivity* (pp. 193–216). Amsterdam: Rodopi.

Frankel, J. (2002). Exploring Ferenczi's concept of identification with the aggressor. *Psychoanalytic Dialogues, 12*(1), 101–139.

Freud, A. (1967). *The ego and the mechanisms of defense* (Rev. ed.). New York: International Universities Press.

Freud, S. (1900). *The interpretation of dreams.* London: Hogarth Press.

Freud, S. (1910). Letter from Sigmund Freud to C. G. Jung, February 2, 1910. In W. McGuire (Ed.), *The Freud/Jung letters* (pp. 290–293). Princeton, NJ: Princeton University Press.

Freud, S. (1912). Recommendations to physicians practicing psychoanalysis. In J. Strachey (Ed. & Trans.), *The standard edition of the complete psychological works of Sigmund Freud* (Vol. 12, pp. 109–120). London: Hogarth Press.

Freud, S. (1920). A child is being beaten: A contribution to the study of the origin of sexual perversions. *International Journal of Psychoanalysis, 1*, 371–395.

Freud, S. (1925). Negation. *International Journal of Psychoanalysis, 6,* 235–239.
Freud, S. (1928). *The future of an illusion.* New York: H. Liveright.
Freud, S. (1952). *The case of Dora.* New York: W. W. Norton.
Freud, S. (1953). The unconscious. In J. Strachey (Ed. & Trans.), *The standard edition of the complete psychological works of Sigmund Freud* (Vol. 14, pp. 161–215). London: Hogarth Press. (Original work published 1915)
Freud, S., Fichtner, G., & Binswanger, L. (2003). *The Sigmund Freud–Ludwig Binswanger correspondence 1908–1938.* New York: Other Press.
Frie, R. (2008). *Psychological agency: Theory, practice, and culture.* Cambridge, MA: MIT Press.
Frie, R., & Orange, D. M. (2009). *Beyond postmodernism: New dimensions in theory and practice.* London: Routledge.
Friedman, L. (2000). Modern hermeneutics and psychoanalysis. *Psychoanalytic Quarterly, 69*(2), 225–264.
Fromm-Reichmann, F. (1950). *Principles of intensive psychotherapy.* Chicago: University of Chicago Press.
Fromm-Reichmann, F. (1954). Psychoanalytic and general dynamic conceptions of theory and of therapy: Differences and similarities. *Journal of the American Psychoanalytic Association, 2,* 711–721.
Fromm-Reichmann, F. (1955a). Clinical significance of intuitive processes of the psychoanalyst. *Journal of the American Psychoanalytic Association, 3,* 82–88.
Fromm-Reichmann, F. (1955b). Intuitive processes in the psychotherapy of schizophrenics: Introduction. *Journal of the American Psychoanalytic Association, 3,* 5–6.
Fromm-Reichmann, F. (1959). *Psychoanalysis and psychotherapy: Selected papers.* Chicago: University of Chicago Press.
Fromm-Reichmann, F. (1990). Loneliness. *Contemporary Psychoanalysis, 26,* 305–329.
Fromm-Reichmann, F., & Silver, A. S. (1990). The assets of the mentally handicapped. *Journal of the American Academy of Psychoanalysis, 18*(1), 47–72.
Fryer, D. (2007). What Lévinas and psychoanalysis can teach each other: Or how to be a mensche without going meshugah. *Psychoanalytic Review, 94,* 577–594.
Gabbard, G. O., & Scarfone, D. (2002). "Controversial discussions": The issue of differences in method. *International Journal of Psychoanalysis, 83*(2), 453–456.
Gadamer, H.-G. (1976). *Philosophical hermeneutics.* Berkeley: University of California Press.

Gadamer, H.-G. (1979a). The problem of historical consciousness. In P. Rabinow & W. Sullivan (Eds.), *Interpretive social science: A reader* (pp. 103–163). Berkeley: University of California Press.

Gadamer, H.-G. (1979b). Practical philosophy as a model of the human sciences. *Research in Phenomenology*, 9, 74–85.

Gadamer, H.-G. (1982). *Reason in the age of science*. Cambridge, MA: MIT Press.

Gadamer, H.-G. (1984). The hermeneutics of suspicion. In G. Shapiro & A. Sica (Eds.), *Hermeneutics: Questions and prospects* (pp. 54–65). Amherst: University of Massachusetts Press.

Gadamer, H.-G. (1987). *Die Universität Heidelberg und die Geburt der modernen Wissenschaft*. New York: Springer-Verlag.

Gadamer, H.-G. (1993). Selbstdarstellung Hans-Georg Gadamer. In *Gesammelte Werke* (Vol. 2, pp. 479–508). Tübingen: Mohr Siebeck. (Original work published 1973)

Gadamer, H.-G. (1996). *The enigma of health: The art of healing in a scientific age*. Stanford, CA: Stanford University Press.

Gadamer, H.-G., Dutt, C., & Palmer, R. E. (2001). *Gadamer in conversation: Reflections and commentary*. New Haven, CT: Yale University Press.

Gadamer, H.-G., & Hahn, L. E. (1997). *The philosophy of Hans-Georg Gadamer*. Chicago: Open Court.

Gadamer, H.-G., & Silverman, H. J. (1991). *Gadamer and hermeneutics*. New York; London: Routledge.

Gadamer, H.-G., Weinsheimer, J., & Marshall, D. G. (2004). *Truth and method* (2nd rev. ed.). New York: Continuum.

Gedo, J. E. (1996). Tribute to a serious man. *The Annual of Psychoanalysis*, 24, 35–40.

Ghent, E. (1990). Masochism, submission, surrender: Masochism as a perversion of surrender. *Contemporary Psychoanalysis*, 26, 108–136.

Gladwell, M. (2008). *Outliers: The story of success*. New York: Little, Brown.

Goldman, D. (1998). Surviving as scientist and dreamer: Winnicott and "The use of an object." *Contemporary Psychoanalysis*, 34(3), 359–367.

Goleman, D. (1995). *Emotional intelligence*. New York: Bantam Books.

Gonzalez, F. (2006). Dialectic and dialogue in the hermeneutics of Paul Ricoeur and H. G. Gadamer. *Continental Philosophy Review*, 39, 313–345.

Gotthold, J. (2009). Peeling the onion: Understanding layers of treatment. In N. VanDerHeide & W. J. Coburn (Eds.), *Self and systems: Explorations in contemporary self psychology* (Vol. 1159, pp. 301–312). New York: New York Academy of Sciences.

Green, H. (1967). "In praise of my doctor": Frieda Fromm-Reichmann. *Contemporary Psychoanalysis, 4*(1), 73–77.

Greenberg, J. (1964). *I never promised you a rose garden: A novel*. New York: Henry Holt.

Greenberg, J. R., & Mitchell, S. A. (1983). *Object relations in psychoanalytic theory*. Cambridge, MA: Harvard University Press.

Greenfield, B., & Jensen, G. (2010). Understanding the lived experiences of patients: The application of phenomenological approach to ethics. *Physical Therapy, 90*, 1–14.

Grondin, J. (1994). *Introduction to philosophical hermeneutics*. New Haven, CT: Yale University Press.

Grondin, J., & Weinsheimer, J. (2003). *Hans-Georg Gadamer: A biography*. New Haven, CT: Yale University Press.

Gump, J. P. (2000). A White therapist, an African American patient: Shame in the therapeutic dyad. *Psychoanalytic Dialogues, 10*(4), 619–632.

Gump, J. P. (2010). Reality matters: The shadow of trauma on African American subjectivity. *Psychoanalytic Psychology, 27*, 42–54.

Guntrip, H. (1996). My experience of analysis with Fairbairn and Winnicott. *International Journal of Psychoanalysis, 77*, 739–754.

Habermas, J. (1953, July 25). Mit Heidegger gegen Heidegger denken. Zur Veröffentlichung von Vorlesungen aus dem Jahre 1935. *Frankfurter Allgemeine Zeitung*.

Habermas, J. (1971). *Knowledge and human interests*. Boston: Beacon Press.

Harris, A. (2009). The socio-political recruitment of identities. *Psychoanalytic Dialogues, 19*, 138–147.

Harris, A., & Aron, L. (1997). Ferenczi's semiotic theory: Previews of postmodernism. *Psychoanalytic Inquiry, 17*(4), 522–534.

Harris, A., & Gold, B. H. (2001). The fog rolled in. *Psychoanalytic Dialogue, 11*(3), 357–384.

Hart, O. V. D., Nijenhuis, E. R. S., & Steele, K. (2006). *The haunted self: Structural dissociation and the treatment of chronic traumatization*. New York: W. W. Norton.

Haynal, A. (1989a). The concept of trauma and its present meaning. *International Review of Psychoanalysis, 16*, 315–321.

Haynal, A. (1989b). *Controversies in psychoanalytic method: From Freud and Ferenczi to Michael Balint*. New York: New York University Press.

Haynal, A. (1992). Introduction to *The correspondence of Sigmund Freud and Sándor Ferenczi*. In E. Brabant, E. Falzeder, & P. Giampieri-Deutsch (Eds.), *The correspondence of Sigmund Freud and Sándor Ferenczi Volume 1, 1908–1914* (pp. xvii–xxxv). Cambridge, MA: Harvard University Press.

Haynal, A. (1993). *Psychoanalysis and the sciences: Epistemology—History*. Berkeley: University of California Press.

Haynal, A. E., & Falzeder, E. (1993). Empathy, psychoanalytic practice in the 1920s, and Ferenczi's "Clinical Diary." *Journal of the American Academy of Psychoanalysis*, 21(4), 605–621.

Heidegger, M. (1962). *Being and time*. London: SCM Press.

Heidegger, M., & Boss, M. (2001). *Zollikon seminars: Protocols, conversations, letters*. Evanston, IL: Northwestern University Press.

Hirsch, I. (1998). The concept of enactment and theoretical convergence. *Psychoanalytic Quarterly*, 67(1), 78–101.

Hoffer, A. (1991). The Freud–Ferenczi controversy: A living legacy. *International Review of Psychoanalysis*, 18, 465–472.

Hoffer, A. (1996). Introduction to *The correspondence of Sigmund Freud and Sándor Ferenczi*. In E. Falzeder, E. Brabant, & P. Giampieri-Deutsch (Eds.), *The correspondence of Sigmund Freud and Sándor Ferenczi Volume 2, 1914–1919* (pp. xvii–xlvi). Cambridge, MA: Harvard University Press.

Hoffer, P. T., & Hoffer, A. (1999). Ferenczi's fatal illness in historical context. *Journal of the American Psychoanalytic Association*, 47(4), 1257–1268.

Hoffman, I. Z. (1994). Dialectical thinking and therapeutic action in the psychoanalytic process. *Psychoanalytic Quarterly*, 63, 187–218.

Hoffman, I. Z. (2009a). Doublethinking our way to "scientific" legitimacy: The desiccation of human experience. *Journal of the American Psychoanalytic Association*, 57, 1043–1069.

Hoffman, I. Z. (2009b). Therapeutic passion in the countertransference. *Psychoanalytic Dialogues*, 19, 617–637.

Hoffmann, K. (1998). Frieda Fromm-Reichmann. *International Forum of Psychoanalysis*, 7(2), 85–96.

Hopkins, B. (1997). Winnicott and the capacity to believe. *International Journal of Psychoanalysis*, 78, 485–497.

Hopkins, L. B. (1998). D. W. Winnicott's analysis of Masud Khan: A preliminary study of failures of object usage. *Contemporary Psychoanalysis*, 34(1), 5–47.

Hornstein, G. A. (2000). *To redeem one person is to redeem the world: The life of Frieda Fromm-Reichmann*. New York: Free Press.

Hutchens, B. (2007). Is Lévinas relevant to psychoanalysis? *Psychoanalytic Review, 94,* 595–616.

Hycner, R., & Jacobs, L. (1995). *The healing relationship in gestalt therapy.* Orleans, MA: Gestalt Therapy Press.

Institute for Contemporary Psychoanalysis. (2010). Dr. Brandchaft book celebration program. Los Angeles, CA. May 16.

Irigaray, L., & Whitford, M. (1991). *The Irigaray reader.* Cambridge, MA: Basil Blackwell.

Jacobs, L. (2010). Speaking evocatively: Prose and wisdom of Erv and Miriam Polster. *Gestalt Review, 14,* 2.

Jaenicke, C. (2008). *The risk of relatedness: Intersubjectivity theory in clinical practice.* Lanham, MD: Jason Aronson.

Jaenicke, C. (2011). *Change in psychoanalysis: An analyst's reflections on the therapeutic relationship.* New York: Routledge.

Jones, E. (1961). *The life and work of Sigmund Freud.* New York: Basic Books.

Josselson, R. (2004). The hermeneutics of faith and the hermeneutics of suspicion. *Narrative Inquiry, 14,* 1–29.

Kahr, B. (1996). *D. W. Winnicott: A biographical portrait.* Madison, CT: International Universities Press.

Kahr, B. (2003). Masud Khan's analysis with Donald Winnicott: On the hazards of befriending a patient. *Free Associations, 10,* 190–222.

Khan, M. R. (1963). The concept of cumulative trauma. *The Psychoanalytic Study of the Child, 18,* 286–306.

Kilborne, B. (1999). Shame in context. *Journal of the American Psychoanalytic Association, 47*(3), 949–952.

Kohut, H. (1959). Introspection, empathy, and psychoanalysis: An examination of the relationship between mode of observation and theory. *Journal of the American Psychoanalytic Association, 7,* 459–483.

Kohut, H. (1971). *The analysis of the self: A systematic approach to the psychoanalytic treatment of narcissistic personality disorders.* New York: International Universities Press.

Kohut, H. (1972). Thoughts on narcissism and narcissistic rage. *The Psychoanalytic Study of the Child, 27,* 360–400.

Kohut, H. (1975). The future of psychoanalysis. *The Annual of Psychoanalysis, 3,* 325–340.

Kohut, H. (1977). *The restoration of the self.* New York: International Universities Press.

Kohut, H. (1979). The two analyses of Mr. Z. *International Journal of Psychoanalysis, 60,* 3–27.

Kohut, H. (1982). Introspection, empathy, and the semi-circle of mental health. *International Journal of Psychoanalysis, 63*, 395–407.

Kohut, H. (1985). On courage. In C. Strozier & E. Kohut (Eds.), *Self psychology and the humanities* (pp. 5–50). New York: Norton.

Kohut, H., Goldberg, A., & Stepansky, P. E. (1984). *How does analysis cure?* Chicago: University of Chicago Press.

Kohut, H., & Ornstein, P. H. (1978). *The search for the self: Selected writings of Heinz Kohut, 1950–1978*. New York: International Universities Press.

Kohut, H., Tolpin, P., & Tolpin, M. (1996). *Heinz Kohut: The Chicago Institute lectures*. Hillsdale, NJ: Analytic Press.

Kraemer, S. B. (1996). "Betwixt the dark and the daylight" of maternal subjectivity: Meditations on the threshold. *Psychoanalytic Dialogues, 6*(6), 765–791.

Kuhn, T. S. (1962). *The structure of scientific revolutions*. Chicago: University of Chicago Press.

Kunz, G. (1998). *The paradox of power and weakness: Lévinas and an alternative paradigm for psychology*. Albany: State University of New York Press.

Lachmann, F. M. (2008). *Transforming narcissism: Reflections on empathy, humor, and expectations*. New York: Analytic Press.

Lansky, M. R. (1994). Shame. *Journal of the American Academy of Psychoanalysis, 22*(3), 433–441.

Lear, J. (2006). *Radical hope: Ethics in the face of cultural devastation*. Cambridge, MA: Harvard University Press.

Lévinas, E. (1969). *Totality and infinity: An essay on exteriority*. Pittsburgh, PA: Duquesne University Press.

Lévinas, E. (1981). *Otherwise than being: Or, beyond essence*. The Hague: the Netherlands: M. Nijhoff.

Lévinas, E. (1990). *Difficult freedom: Essays on Judaism*. Baltimore: Johns Hopkins University Press.

Lévinas, E. (1996). *Proper names*. Stanford, CA: Stanford University Press.

Lévinas, E. (1998a). *Entre nous: On thinking-of-the-other*. New York: Columbia University Press.

Lévinas, E. (1998b). *Of God who comes to mind* (2nd ed.). Stanford, CA: Stanford University Press.

Lévinas, E., & Nemo, P. (1985). *Ethics and infinity*. Pittsburgh, PA: Duquesne University Press.

Lévinas, E., Peperzak, A. T., Critchley, S., & Bernasconi, R. (1996). *Emmanuel Lévinas: Basic philosophical writings*. Bloomington: Indiana University Press.

Lévinas, E., & Robbins, J. (2001). *Is it righteous to be? Interviews with Emmanuel Lévinas*. Stanford, CA: Stanford University Press.

Levine, H. B. (1994). Speak of me as I am: The life and work of Masud Khan. *Journal of the American Psychoanalytic Association, 42*, 1286–1290.

Little, M. I. (1990). *Psychotic anxieties and containment: A personal record of an analysis with Winnicott*. Northvale, NJ: Jason Aronson.

Maier-Katkin, D. (2010). *Stranger from abroad: Hannah Arendt, Martin Heidegger, friendship, and forgiveness*. New York: W. W. Norton.

Malka, S. (2006). *Emmanuel Lévinas: His life and legacy*. Pittsburgh, PA: Duquesne University Press.

Margalit, A. (2002). *The ethics of memory*. Cambridge, MA: Harvard University Press.

Maroda, K. (1998a). Enactment. *Psychoanalytic Psychology, 15*(4), 517–535.

Maroda, K. (1998b). Why mutual analysis failed: The case of Ferenczi and RN. *Contemporary Psychoanalysis, 34*(1), 115–132.

McLaughlin, J. T., & Johan, M. (1992). Enactments in psychoanalysis. *Journal of the American Psychoanalytic Association, 40*, 827–841.

Mezaros, J. (2010). Sándor Ferenczi and the Budapest school of psychoanalysis. *Psychoanalytic Perspectives, 7*, 69–89.

Michelfelder, D. P., & Palmer, R. E. (1989). *Dialogue and deconstruction: The Gadamer–Derrida encounter*. Albany: State University of New York Press.

Miller, A. (1979). The drama of the gifted child and the psycho-analyst's narcissistic disturbance. *International Journal of Psychoanalysis, 60*, 47–58.

Mitchell, S. A. (1986). The wings of Icarus: Illusion and the problem of narcissism. *Contemporary Psychoanalysis, 22*, 107–132.

Mitchell, S. A. (2000a). *Relationality: From attachment to intersubjectivity*. Hillsdale, NJ: Analytic Press.

Mitchell, S. A. (2000b). You've got to suffer if you want to sing the blues. *Psychoanalytic Dialogues, 10*(5), 713–733.

Morrison, A. P. (1987). The shame experience. *International Journal of Psychoanalysis, 68*, 307–310.

Morrison, A. P. (1999). Shame in context. *International Journal of Psychoanalysis, 80*(3), 616–619.

Nahum, J. P. (2002). Explicating the implicit. *International Journal of Psychoanalysis, 83*(5), 1051–1062.

Neve, M. (1992). Clare Winnicott talks to Michael Neve. *Free Associations, 3*, 167–184.

Ogden, T. H. (1982). *Projective identification and psychotherapeutic technique*. New York: Jason Aronson.
Ogden, T. H. (2001). Reading Winnicott. *Psychoanalytic Quarterly, 70*(2), 299–323.
Ogden, T. H. (2003). What's true and whose idea was it? *International Journal of Psychoanalysis, 84*, 593–606.
Orange, D. M. (1995). *Emotional understanding: Studies in psychoanalytic epistemology*. New York: Guilford.
Orange, D. M. (2000). The Chicago Institute lectures. *Psychoanalytic Psychology, 17*(2), 420–431.
Orange, D. M. (2002). There is no outside: Empathy and authenticity in psychoanalytic process. *Psychoanalytic Psychology, 19*, 686–700.
Orange, D. M. (2006). For whom the bell tolls: Context, complexity, and compassion in psychoanalysis. *International Journal of Psychoanalytic Self Psychology, 1*, 5–21.
Orange, D. M. (2008a). Recognition as: Intersubjective vulnerability in the psychoanalytic dialogue. *International Journal of Psychoanalytic Self Psychology, 3*, 178–194.
Orange, D. M. (2008b). Whose shame is it anyway? Lifeworlds of humiliation and systems of restoration. *Contemporary Psychoanalysis, 44*, 83–100.
Orange, D. M. (2009a). Intersubjective systems theory: A fallibilist's journey. In N. VanDerHeide & W. Coburn (Eds.), *Self and systems: Explorations in contemporary self psychology* (pp. 237–248). Boston: Blackwell.
Orange, D. M. (2009b). Kohut memorial lecture: Attitudes, values and intersubjective vulnerability. *International Journal of Psychoanalytic Self Psychology, 4*, 235–253.
Orange, D. M. (2009c). *Thinking for clinicians: Philosophical resources for contemporary psychoanalysis and the humanistic psychotherapies*. New York: Routledge.
Orange, D. M. (2010). Revisiting mutual recognition: Responding to Ringstrom, Benjamin, and Slavin. *International Journal of Psychoanalytic Self Psychology, 5*, 293–306.
Orange, D. M. (2011). Speaking the unspeakable: Traumatic living memory and the dialogue of metaphors. *International Journal of Psychoanalytic Self Psychology, 6*, 187–206.
Orange, D. M., Atwood, G. E., & Stolorow, R. D. (1997). *Working intersubjectively: Contextualism in psychoanalytic practice*. Hillsdale, NJ: Analytic Press.
Ornstein, P. (2005). When "Dora" came to see me for a second analysis. *Psychoanalytic Inquiry, 25*, 94–114.

Palmer, R. (2002). *The relevance of Gadamer's "Philosophical hermeneutics" to thirty-six topics or fields of human activity.* Retrieved from http://www.mac.edu/faculty/richardpalmer/relevance.html

Peirce, C. S. (1931). *Collected papers of Charles Sanders Peirce.* Cambridge, MA: Harvard University Press.

Petratos, B. D. (1990). The European teachers of Dr. Frieda Fromm-Reichmann. *Journal of the American Academy of Psychoanalysis, 18*(1), 152–166.

Phillips, A. (1988). *Winnicott.* Cambridge, MA: Harvard University Press.

Poland, W. S. (2000). The analyst's witnessing and otherness. *Journal of the American Psychoanalytic Association, 48*(1), 17–34.

Poland, W. S. (2001). Controversial discussions. *Journal of the American Psychoanalytic Association, 49*(2), 347–354.

Rachman, A. W. (1997a). Sándor Ferenczi and the evolution of a self psychology framework in psychoanalysis. *Progress in Self Psychology, 13*, 341–365.

Rachman, A. W. (1997b). The suppression and censorship of Ferenczi's "Confusion of tongues" paper. *Psychoanalytic Inquiry, 17*(4), 459–485.

Racker, H. (1968). *Transference and counter-transference.* New York: International Universities Press.

Reeder, J. (1998). Hermeneutics and intersubjectivity. *International Forum of Psychoanalysis, 7*(2), 65–75.

Ricoeur, P. (1970). *Freud and philosophy: An essay on interpretation.* New Haven, CT: Yale University Press.

Ricoeur, P. (1992). *Oneself as another.* Chicago: University of Chicago Press.

Risser, J. (1997). *Hermeneutics and the voice of the other.* Albany: State University of New York Press.

Roazen, P. (1975). *Freud and his followers.* New York: Knopf.

Roazen, P. (1997). Brett Kahr. D. W. Winnicott: A biographical portrait. *International Forum of Psychoanalysis, 6*(3), 207–208.

Roazen, P. (2001a). The controversial discussions. *International Forum of Psychoanalysis, 10*(3–4), 259–274.

Roazen, P. (2001b). *The historiography of psychoanalysis.* New Brunswick, NJ: Transaction Publishers.

Rodman, F. R. (2003). *Winnicott: Life and work.* Cambridge, MA: Perseus.

Rowling, J. K. (2000). *Harry Potter and the goblet of fire* (1st American ed.). New York: Arthur A. Levine Books.

Rozmarin, E. (2007). An other in psychoanalysis. *Contemporary Psychoanalysis, 43*, 327–360.

Rozmarin, E. (2010). Better identity politics. *Psychoanalytic Dialogues, 20*, 181–190.

Rudnytsky, P. L. (2002). *Reading psychoanalysis: Freud, Rank, Ferenczi, Groddeck*. Ithaca, NY: Cornell University Press.

Rudnytsky, P. L., Bókay, A., & Giampieri-Deutsch, P. (1996). *Ferenczi's turn in psychoanalysis*. New York: New York University Press.

Safranski, R. (1998). *Martin Heidegger: Between good and evil*. Cambridge, MA: Harvard University Press.

Sander, L. W. (1988). The event-structure of regulation in the neonate-caregiver system as a biological background for early organization of psychic structure. *Progress in Self Psychology, 3*, 64–77.

Sander, L. W. (2002). Thinking differently. *Psychoanalytic Dialogues, 12*(1), 11–42.

Sartre, J.-P. (2001). *Being and nothingness*. New York: Citadel Press.

Sass, L. A. (1989). Humanism, hermeneutics, and humanistic psychoanalysis: Differing conceptions of subjectivity. *Psychoanalysis and Contemporary Thought, 12*, 433–504.

Schleiermacher, F., & Bowie, A. (1998). *Hermeneutics and criticism and other writings*. Cambridge, UK: Cambridge University Press.

Schleiermacher, F., & Kimmerle, H. (1977). *Hermeneutics: The handwritten manuscripts*. Missoula, MT: Scholars Press for the American Academy of Religion.

Schleiermacher, F., & Schmidt, G. G. (2001). *Letters on the occasion of the political theological task and the Sendschreiben (open letter) of Jewish heads of households*. Lewiston, NY: Edwin Mellen Press.

Schürmann, R., Critchley, S., & Levine, S. (2008). *On Heidegger's* Being and time. London: Routledge.

Searles, H. (1975). The patient as therapist to his analyst. *Countertransference and related subjects* (pp. 380–459). New York: International Universities Press.

Shaw, D. (2003). On the therapeutic action of analytic love. *Contemporary Psychoanalysis, 39*, 251–278.

Shengold, L. (1979). Child abuse and deprivation soul murder. *Journal of the American Psychoanalytic Association, 27*, 533–559.

Shengold, L. (1989). *Soul murder: The effects of childhood abuse and deprivation*. New Haven, CT: Yale University Press.

Siegel, A. M. (1996). *Heinz Kohut and the psychology of the self*. London: Routledge.

Silver, A. (1993). Countertransference, Ferenczi, and Washington, DC. *Journal of the American Academy of Psychoanalysis, 21*, 637–654.

Silver, A. S. (1992). Treating the hospitalized borderline patient. *Journal of the American Academy of Psychoanalysis, 20*(1), 114–129.

Silver, A. S. (1996). Frieda Fromm-Reichmann, loneliness and deafness. *International Forum of Psychoanalysis, 5*(1), 39–45.

Silver, A. S. (1999). Frieda Fromm-Reichmann and Erich Fromm. *International Forum of Psychoanalysis, 8*(1), 19–23.

Silver, A. S., & Fromm-Reichmann, F. (1989). *Psychoanalysis and psychosis*. Madison, CT: International Universities Press.

Slochower, J. A. (1998). Illusion and uncertainty in psychoanalytic writing. *International Journal of Psychoanalysis, 79*, 333–347.

Spence, D. P. (1982). *Narrative truth and historical truth: Meaning and interpretation in psychoanalysis*. New York; London: W. W. Norton.

Staemmler, F.-M. (2007). The willingness to be uncertain: Preliminary thoughts about interpretation and understanding in gestalt therapy. *International Gestalt Journal, 29*, 11–42.

Staemmler, F.-M. (2009). *Das Geheimnis des Anderen: Empathie in der Psychotherapie aus neuer Perspektive*. Stuttgart: Klett-Cotta.

Stanton, M. (1991). *Sándor Ferenczi: Reconsidering active intervention*. Northvale, NJ: Jason Aronson.

Steele, R. S. (1979). Psychoanalysis and hermeneutics. *International Review of Psychoanalysis, 6*, 389–411.

Steiner, R. (1995). Hermeneutics or hermes-mess? *International Journal of Psychoanalysis, 76*, 435–445.

Stern, D. B. (1997). *Unformulated experience: From dissociation to imagination in psychoanalysis*. Hillsdale, NJ: Analytic Press.

Stern, D. B. (2009). *Partners in thought: Working with unformulated experience, dissociation, and enactment*. New York: Routledge.

Stern, D. N. (1985). *The interpersonal world of the infant*. New York: Basic Books.

Stevenson, B. E. (1998). Silenced women, personal art, and motherhood. *Psychoanalytic Inquiry, 18*(2), 183–192.

Stolorow, R. D. (2007). *Trauma and human existence: Autobiographical, psychoanalytic, and philosophical reflections*. New York: Analytic Press.

Stolorow, R. D., & Atwood, G. E. (1984). Psychoanalytic phenomenology: Toward a science of human experience. *Psychoanalytic Inquiry, 4*(1), 87–105.

Stolorow, R. D., & Atwood, G. E. (1992). *Contexts of being: The intersubjective foundations of psychological life*. Hillsdale, NJ: Analytic Press.

Stolorow, R. D., & Atwood, G. E. (1996). The intersubjective perspective. *Psychoanalytic Review, 83*(2), 181–194.

Stolorow, R. D., Atwood, G. E., & Brandchaft, B. (1987). *Psychoanalytic treatment: An intersubjective approach*. Hillsdale, NJ: Analytic Press.

Stolorow, R. D., Atwood, G. E., & Brandchaft, B. (1994). *The intersubjective perspective*. Northvale, NJ: Jason Aronson.

Stolorow, R. D., Atwood, G. E., & Orange, D. M. (1999). Kohut and contextualism. *Psychoanalytic Psychology, 16*(3), 380–388.

Stolorow, R. D., Atwood, G. E., & Orange, D. M. (2002). *Worlds of experience: Interweaving philosophical and clinical dimensions in psychoanalysis*. New York: Basic Books.

Stolorow, R. D., Atwood, G. E., & Orange, D. M. (2010). Heidegger's Nazism and the hypostatization of being. *International Journal of Psychoanalytic Self Psychology, 5*(4), 429–450.

Straker, G. (2007). A crisis in the subjectivity of the analyst: The trauma of morality. *Psychoanalytic Dialogues, 17*, 153–164.

Suchet, M. (2010). Face to face. *Psychoanalytic Dialogues, 20*, 158–171.

Suttie, I. D. (1988). *The origins of love and hate*. London: Free Association Books.

Szalita, A. B. (1981). Acceptance speech on the occasion of receiving the Frieda Fromm-Reichmann award. *Journal of the American Academy of Psychoanalysis, 9*(1), 11–16.

Szalita, A. B. (2001). Some thoughts on empathy. *Contemporary Psychoanalysis, 37*(1), 95–111.

Tähkä, R. (2000). Illusion and reality in the psychoanalytic relationship. *Scandinavian Psychoanalytic Review, 23*(1), 65–88.

Turner, J. F. (2002). A brief history of illusion. *International Journal of Psychoanalysis, 83*(5), 1063–1082.

Usuelli, A. K. (1992). The significance of illusion in the work of Freud and Winnicott: A controversial issue. *International Review of Psycho-Analysis, 19*, 179–187.

Vida, J. (1993). Ferenczi's clinical diary: Roadmap to the realm of primary relatedness. *Journal of the American Academy of Psychoanalysis, 21*(4), 623–635.

Vida, J. E. (1996). The "wise baby" grows up: The contemporary relevance of Sándor Ferenczi. In P. Rudnytsky, A. Bokay, & P. Giamieri-Deutsch (Eds.), *Ferenczi's turn in psychoanalysis*. New York: New York University Press, 266–286.

Vida, J. E. (1997). The voice of Ferenczi: Echoes from the past. *Psychoanalytic Inquiry, 17*(4), 404–415.

Vida, J. E. (1999). Considering androgyny. *International Forum of Psychoanalysis, 8*(3–4), 257–262.

Vida, J. E. (2001). Ferenczi's "teratoma." *International Forum of Psychoanalysis, 10*(3–4), 235–241.

Vida, J. E., & Molad, G. (2004). The Ferenczian dialogue: Psychoanalysis as a way of life. *Free Associations, 11*, 338–352.

Wachterhauser, B. (2002). Getting it right: Relativism, realism, and truth. In R. Dostal (Ed.), *The Cambridge companion to Gadamer* (pp. 52–78). Cambridge, UK: Cambridge University Press.

Warnke, G. (1987). *Gadamer: Hermeneutics, tradition, and reason.* Oxford: Polity Press.

Winnicott, D. W. (1941). The observation of infants in a set situation. *International Journal of Psychoanalysis, 22*, 229–249.

Winnicott, D. W. (1945). Primitive emotional development. *International Journal of Psychoanalysis, 26*, 137–143.

Winnicott, D. W. (1949). Hate in the countertransference. *International Journal of Psychoanalysis, 30*, 69–74.

Winnicott, D. W. (1953). Transitional objects and transitional phenomena: A study of the first not-me possession. *International Journal of Psychoanalysis, 34*, 89–97.

Winnicott, D. W. (1955). Metapsychological and clinical aspects of regression within the psycho-analytical set-up. *International Journal of Psychoanalysis, 36*, 16–26.

Winnicott, D. W. (1958a). The capacity to be alone. *International Journal of Psychoanalysis, 39*, 416–420.

Winnicott, D. W. (1958b). *Collected papers: Through paediatrics to psycho-analysis.* New York: Basic Books.

Winnicott, D. W. (1960). The theory of the parent–infant relationship. *International Journal of Psychoanalysis, 41*, 585–595.

Winnicott, D. W. (1963). Dependence in infant care, in child care, and in the psycho-analytic setting. *International Journal of Psychoanalysis, 44*, 339–344.

Winnicott, D. W. (1965). *The maturational processes and the facilitating environment: Studies in the theory of emotional development.* New York: International Universities Press.

Winnicott, D. W. (1967). The location of cultural experience. *International Journal of Psychoanalysis, 48*, 368–372.

Winnicott, D. W. (1968). Playing: Its theoretical status in the clinical situation. *International Journal of Psychoanalysis, 49*, 591–599.

Winnicott, D. W. (1969). The use of an object. *International Journal of Psychoanalysis, 50*, 711–716.

Winnicott, D. W. (1971). *Playing and reality.* New York: Basic Books.

Winnicott, D. W. (1974). Fear of breakdown. *International Review of Psychoanalysis, 1*, 103–107.

Winnicott, D. W. (1977). *The piggle: An account of the psychoanalytic treatment of a little girl.* New York: International University Press.

Winnicott, D. W. (1992). *Through paediatrics to psycho-analysis: Collected papers.* New York: Brunner/Mazel.

Winnicott, D. W., Winnicott, C., Shepherd, R., & Davis, M. (1986). *Home is where we start from: Essays by a psychoanalyst.* New York: Norton.

Winnicott, D. W., Winnicott, C., Shepherd, R., & Davis, M. (1989). *Psychoanalytic explorations.* Cambridge, MA: Harvard University Press.

Wittgenstein, L. (1953). *Philosophical investigations.* New York: Macmillan.

Wolf, E. S. (1988). *Treating the self: Elements of clinical self psychology.* New York: Guilford.

Wolf, E. S. (1997). Self psychology and the aging self throughout the life curve. *The Annual of Psychoanalysis, 25,* 201–215.

Yalom, I. D. (1980). *Existential psychotherapy.* New York: Basic Books.

Yalom, I. D. (2008). *Staring at the sun: Overcoming the terror of death.* San Francisco, CA: Jossey-Bass.

Young-Bruehl, E. (2002). A visit to the Budapest school. *The Psychoanalytic Study of the Child, 57,* 411–432.

Young-Eisendrath, P. (2001). When the fruit ripens. *Psychoanalytic Quarterly, 70*(1), 265–285.

Index

A

Accommodation
  hermeneutics of pathological, 218–224
  pathological, 68
Active techniques, 78
Agency, 51–52, 66–67
Aloneness, 129–130. *See also* Loneliness
Alterity, 53
Analytic process, sloppiness of, 194
Annihilation, 150–151
Antiquity, adhering to the dictates of, 219–220
Anxiety
  clinical relationships and, 129–130
  developmental origins of, 120–121
Asymmetric role responsibility, intersubjectivity and, 109
Asymmetry, 57
Attachment, survival and, 226
Attitude of receptivity, 67–68
Attunement, 192–193
Atwood, George, 208–209, 215
Authenticity, 51–52, 168

B

Befindlichkeit, 59
Behandlung, 39
Belonging, 32–33, 47
Benefit of the doubt, 64–65
Bion, Wilfred, 208
Bonhoeffer, Dietrich, 135
Boston Process of Change Study Group, 192–194
Boundaries, 131–135
Brandchaft, Bernard, 183
  life and work of, 206–209
  obsessionality and the hermeneutics of trust, 228–233
  systems of pathological accommodation, 68, 76, 93–94, 148, 214–228
Breakdowns
  fear of, 144, 154–155
  Winnicott's understanding of, 149

Buber, Martin, 117
Bullard, Dexter, 117

C

Capacity, Winnicott's ideas on, 145–146
Categorizing, 61
Chestnut Lodge, 116–117
Child analysis in the analysis of adults, 108. *See also* Ferenczi, Sándor
Childhood trauma. *See also* Ferenczi, Sándor
 Ferenczi's theory of teratoma due to, 95–97
Classifying, 46, 61
Clinical hermeneutics
 Ferenczi's practice of, 79, 103–106
 Fromm-Reichmann's practice of, 123–125
 Winnicott's practice of, 162–165
Compassion, 188
Compassion fatigue, 108
Complexity, 10, 203
 hermeneutics of, 156–162
 Kohut's views on, 195–198
Complexity of significance, 143–145
Compliance, Winnicott's interpretation of, 148–149
Confusion of tongues, 88–94, 226, 231
Contextualism, 202
Contrite fallibilism, 173, 203, 213–214
Conversation, 15–16, 19–20, 41
 interpretation and, 21
 relational psychoanalysis and, 22–23
Countertransference, 59, 77, 122–123, 129
 Winnicott's thoughts on, 141
Cumulative trauma, 93–94

D

Defenses, 97, 105, 153, 183
 hermeneutics of, 209–215
Dependency, 76
 hermeneutics of, 149–154
Development
 hermeneutics of, 145–146
 intersubjective systems theory of, 215–218 (*See also* Intersubjective systems theory)
 pathological accommodation and, 223–224
Developmental hermeneutics, 191–202
Developmental second chance, 153–154
Developmentalists, misattunements and, 193–194
Dialogical hermeneutics, 3, 33–35, 41, 206. *See also* Gadamer, Hans-Georg
 equilibrium and, 21–22
 Fromm-Reichmann and, 111–112
 trust in, 43–45
Dialogical understanding, 17–18
Dilthey, Wilhelm, 12–13
Disappearing interpretation, 20–21, 134
Disappointment, developmental necessity of, 202
Disintegration products, 189
Disruption, 62–63
Dissociative freezing, 128, 152
Double guile, 27
Double reading, 167–168
Dream interpretation, 28–29
Dream of the learned infant, 84–85. *See also* Wise baby
Dynamic unconsciousness, origin of, 121

E

Eigenbedeutsamkeit, 17
Einfuhlung, 178
Emancipatory psychoanalysis, 215, 224
Empathic attunement, 192–193
Empathy, 8, 176
    Kohut's texts concerning, 183–184
    Kohut's understanding of, 178–183
    responding to others' needs and, 186
Enactments, 67
Erasure, 54
Esotericism, 30
Ethical relation of proximity, 48
Ethics, 46, 59
Ethics of humanism, 203–204
Evidence-based treatment, 9
Experience-near language, 57
Extraterritoriality, 53

F

Face, 61
    concept of, 45–46
Face of the suffering stranger, 45–54
Facial changes, psychoanalysts' perceptions and, 183–184
Failure, 231–233
    freezing of, 151
Faith and restoration, hermeneutics of, 31–32
Fallibilism, 24, 194, 199, 208
    contrite, 173, 203, 213–214
False self, 148
    pathological accommodation and, 221–222
Fear of breakdown, 154–155
    Winnicott's concept of, 144
Ferenczi, Sándor, 74, 115–116, 131, 149, 153, 178–179, 187, 231
    "Confusion of Tongues" paper, 80, 88–94
    active techniques of, 78
    analytic attitude of, 98–101
    clinical attitudes of, 107–109
    hermeneutics of, 82–84, 86–88
    hubris of, 171
    life and work of, 76–82
    mutual analysis method, 79
    relaxation method, 79
Finitude, 23–24
First philosophy, 46
Flexible therapeutic boundaries, trust and, 131–135
Fore-understanding, 14
Fragmentation, 189
Free aggressivity, 189–191
Freedom, 51–52
Freezing, 128
Freud, Anna, reaction of to Kohut's self psychology, 176
Freud, Sigmund, 2, 26, 73, 114, 205, 210
    final dispute with Ferenczi, 89
    hermeneutics of suspicion, 26–31, 34–35
    hubris of, 171–172
Freud–Ferenczi correspondence, 75
Freudian psychoanalysis, 4
Fromm, Erich, 116
Fromm-Reichmann, Frieda
    clinical sensibility of, 123–125
    hermeneutics of, 118–123
    life and work of, 111–118
    therapeutic boundaries and trust, 131–135
    understanding of hermeneutics of loneliness, 125–131
Frozen failure, 151
Furor sanandi, 101
Fusion of horizons, 41

G

Gadamer, Hans-Georg, 3, 14–22
    hermeneutics of trust, 32–35

Gadamerian hermeneutics, 14–22
    Lévinasian hospitality and, 60–66
Gestalt psychology, 60, 115
Ghent, Emmanuel, 163
    concept of surrender, 23, 52,
        67–68
Goldstein, Kurt, 115
Good-enough mother, 160
    true self and, 148
Gourevitch, Anna, 123
Grammatical hermeneutics, 6
Grandiose patients, Lévinasian
        therapeutics and, 57–58
Greenberg, Joanne, 117, 133–135
Groddeck, Georg, 78, 115–116
Guilt, 66

H

Hate
    development of the true self and,
        169–170
    relational causality of, 181
    Winnicott's ideas of, 142–143
Heidegger, Martin, 3, 13–14, 168
    hubris of, 171
Helpful doctor, 83
Hermeneutic circle, 10, 13, 16, 32
    Fromm-Reichmann's form of,
        119–120
    Kohut's form of, 198
    use of to approach Winnicott's
        writings, 142
Hermeneutic clinical sensibility,
    25–26
Hermeneutic phenomenology, 14
Hermeneutic psychoanalysis,
        Ferenczi's practice of, 79
Hermeneutic sensibility, elements of
    in everyday therapeutics,
        22–26
Hermeneutical attitude, 19
Hermeneutics
    Dilthey's contribution to, 12–13
    Fromm-Reichmann's, 118–123

Gadamer's contribution to, 14–22,
    32–33
Gadamer's description of, 40
Heidegger's contribution to,
    13–14
Kohut's, 177–183
origin of, 1–2
Ricoeur's contribution to, 26–31
Schleiermacher's elements of, 6
Winnicott's contribution to,
    141–145
Hermeneutics of complexity,
    156–162
Hermeneutics of defense and
    resistance, Branchaft's
    attitude toward, 209–215
Hermeneutics of dependency,
    149–154
Hermeneutics of development,
    145–146
Hermeneutics of faith and
    restoration of meaning,
    31–32, 205. *See also*
    Hermeneutics of trust
Hermeneutics of incommunicable
    loneliness, 125–131
Hermeneutics of intersubjectivity,
    215–218. *See also*
    Intersubjectivity
Hermeneutics of paradox, 156–162
Hermeneutics of regression, 146–149
Hermeneutics of suffering, Fromm-
    Reichmann's, 118–121
Hermeneutics of suspicion, 26–31,
    73, 160–161, 205
Hermeneutics of trauma, 82–84, 179
    obsessionality and, 228–233
    wise baby, 84–88
Hermeneutics of trust, 31–35, 38–40,
    98–101, 205–206
    clinical practice of, 103–106
    developmental perspectives and,
        191–202
    fear of breakdown and, 154–155

flexible therapeutic boundaries and, 131–135
Fromm-Reichmann's, 122–123
Kohut as practitioner of, 202–204
Kohut's practice of, 182–183
Lévinasian hospitality and, 60–66
practice of, 217
squiggle game as an example of, 138
taking risks and, 184–186
Winnicott's clinical practice and, 165–167
Heroic resistance, 210, 217
Hineni, 49–51
Historicism, 16
Hoffman, Irwin, 172
Hospitality, 55, 65, 153–154
Hubris, dangers of, 171–173
Humanism, ethics of, 203–204
Humanistic psychotherapies, 102
Humility, 203
Husserl, Edmund, 46

I

Identification with the aggressor, 89, 91–93
Illusion
    Freud's view of, 158
    Winnicott's view of, 143, 158–162, 166
Immemorial responsibility, 57–58
Impingement, 150–151
Incarnate subjectivity, 48
Incommunicable loneliness, hermeneutics of, 125–131
Incumbency, 56
Incurable defects, 231–232
Individual subjectivity, 63–64
Infinity, 54, 69
Inner word, 35, 40
Intentionality, 212
Interaction, 67
Internal mother, Winnicott's concept of, 144

Internal objects, 143–144
Interpretation, 14
    disappearing, 20–21
Intersubjective misunderstanding, 89, 193–194
Intersubjective psychoanalysis, 211–215
Intersubjective systems theory, 209, 215–218
    mutuality and, 102
    trauma in, 80
Intersubjectivity, 63, 109, 200–202, 206
    hermeneutics of, 215–218
Intuitive understanding, 6

J

Jones, Ernest, 80–81
    hubris of, 172
Judgment, 56
Jung, Carl, hubris of, 172

K

Khan, Masud, 140, 148, 168
Klein, Melanie, 220–221
    hubris of, 172
Knowledge of the other, 61–62
Kohut, Heinz, 57–58
    developmental hermeneutics of, 191–202
    life and work, 176–177
    practice of hermeneutics of trust by, 202–204
    texts of, 183–191

L

Language
    psychoanalysis and, 22
    use of by Winnicott, 141–144
Learned infant. *See* Wise baby

264 • Index

Lévinas, Emmanuel, 3
  face of the suffering stranger, 45–54
Lévinasian ethic, 108
Lévinasian hospitality, hermeneutics of trust and, 60–66
Lévinasian therapeutics, elements of, 54–60
Little, Margaret, 162
Lived experience, 13
Local level, 192, 194, 200–202
Loneliness
  analysts and, 129–130
  hermeneutics of, 125–131

M

Marx, Karl, 26, 73
Maternal system, 151, 156, 170
Me voici, 47, 49–51
Meaningfulness, 14
Memory, terror as, 154–155
Misattunements, 154, 184
  rupture-and-repair vs., 194–195
Misunderstanding, 5, 193–194
Morality, 59
Mother-infant system, 156
Mutual analysis, 79, 101–103, 109
Mutuality, 57, 199, 216–217

N

Narcissistic patients
  empathy and, 179–180
  Lévinasian therapeutics and, 57–58
  self psychology and, 184–186
Narcissistic rage, 228
  Kohut's rethinking of, 188–191
Negation, 73
Negative transference, 76
Neighbor, 47
Neuroscience, 9
Nietzsche, Friedrich, 26, 73

Nondefensive sincerity, 187. *See also* Sincerity
Nonsurvival, 163
Normal nursery concept, 96–97
Normal science, 205
Nuclear self, 196

O

Objectifications, 188
Obsessional patients, compulsive accommodation of, 218
Obsessionality, rethinking from the hermeneutics of trust, 228–233
Oppression, resistance and, 210
Ornstein, Anna, 175
Ornstein, Paul, 175
Other ego, 46. *See also* The other

P

Paradox, hermeneutics of, 156–162
Parentified child, 87, 164
  Lévinasian therapeutics and, 58–59
Participation, 33
Passion to cure, 101
Pathological accommodation, 68. *See also* Systems of pathological accommodation
  forms of, 224–228
  hermeneutics of, 218–224
  obsessionality and, 231–233
Perceptions, facial changes and, 183–184
Personal agency, 66–67
Personal style, 11
Perspectival realism, 199
Perspective, tradition-formed, 20
Phenomenological hermeneutics, 175, 198
Philosophical hermeneutics, 14–22
Phronesis, 10, 24–25
  hubris and, 172

Possessiveness, 53
Posttraumatic stress, Kohu't early description of, 180
Practical wisdom, 24–25. *See also* Phronesis
Primal failure, 231–232
Principle of charity, 32
Priority of conversation, 15–16
Projection, 14
Proto-fallibilism, 6
Proximity, 157–158
    ethical relation of, 48
Pseudo-psychosis, 180
Psychoanalysis, 4
    defense and resistance in, 209–215
    hermeneutics of suspicion and, 41–42 (*See also* Hermeneutics of suspicion)
    language and, 22
    mutuality of, 101–103
    relational, 22–23
Psychoanalytic witness, 99
Psychological hermeneutics, 7
Psychological trauma. *See also* Trauma
    pathogenesis of, 79–80
Psychopathology, self psychology and, 191–202
Psychosis, empathy and, 189
Psychotherapeutic hospitality, 55
Psychotherapy, relief of suffering and, 66–70

R

Racism, 61
Radical finitude, 24
Rational faith, 31–32
Rationality, 50
Receptive approach, 39, 67–68
Reductionism, 9, 188
Regressed patients, psychoanalysis of, 146–149

Regression
    hermeneutics of, 146–149
    management of, 162–163
Relaxation method, 79
Remembrances, fear of breakdown and, 154–155
Resistance, 64, 183
    hermeneutics of, 209–215
Resoluteness, 168
Responsiveness, 188
Retraumatization, 21, 94, 152, 233
    Ferenczi's view of, 102
    inevitability of, 166
    Kohut's understanding of, 187
Ricoeur, Paul
    hermeneutics of faith, 31–32
    hermeneutics of suspicion, 26–31
    hermeneutics of trust, 51
Rigorous practice, 5–6
Risk avoidance, 230
Rosenfeld, Herbert, 208
Rosenzwieg, Franz, 117
Rules, 131–135
Rupture-and-repair, 189, 200–202
    misattunements *vs.*, 194–195
Ruthlessness, 167
    development of the true self and, 169
    Winnicott's ideas of, 143

S

Sachs, Hans, 115
Schizophrenic patients
    hermeneutics of trust and, 122
    loneliness of, 125–131
    treatment of at Chestnut Lodge, 117
Schleiermacher, Friedrich, 3–12
Scholem, Gershom, 117
School of suspicion, 31, 38. *See also* Hermeneutics of suspicion
Selbstvertrautheit, 5

Self psychology, 175, 180–183
    developmental hermeneutics and,
        191–202
    Kohut's texts on, 183–191
Self-abnegation, 219
Self-hatred, pathological
        accommodation and, 231
Selfobjects, 177
    experience of, 178
Significance, complexity of, 143–145
Sincerity, 103, 173
    nondefensive, 187
Skepticism, 28
Soul murder, 96, 110
Splitting, 95–97
Spoken *vs.* written word, 62
Squiggle game, 7, 138
Stage of ruth, 143
Stolorow, Robert, 208–209
    emancipatory psychoanalysis, 215
Stranger as neighbor, 54–60
Subjection, 52
Subjectivity, 49–50
    incarnate, 48
Subjectivity through subjection, 165
Substitution, 49, 138
Suffering, 23, 68–70
    acceptance of responsibility for,
        100–101
    fear of breakdown and, 154–155
    Fromm-Reichmann's attitudes
        towards, 114–115
    psychotherapy and the relief of,
        66–70
    regression and, 153
Suffering stranger
    Branchaft's response to, 233–235
    Lévinas's face of, 45–54
Sullivan, Harry Stack, 114, 119
Surrender, Ghent's concept of, 23, 52,
        67–68
Survival, 163–164
    attachment and, 226
Suspicion
    forms of, 211
    hermeneutics of, 26–31, 73
Suttie, Ian, 120
Symptoms, meaning in, 124–125
Systems of pathological
        accommodation, 68, 76,
        93–94, 148, 211
Szalita, Alberta, 123

T

Teratoma, 95–97
Terror, 107, 222, 231–233
    as memory, 155
    interpreting, 154–155
Terrorism of suffering, 93–94
The other, 41–43
    knowledge of, 61–62
Therapeutic action, intersubjectivity
        and, 109
Therapeutic boundaries, trust and
        flexibility of, 131–135
Therapeutic process, sloppiness of,
        194
Therapeutic relationship,
        exploitation of, 140–141
Thou shalt nots, 132
Thrown projection, 14
Thrownness, 44, 168
Tolpin, Marian, 175
Total self, 196
Totalizing, 46, 54
Tradition, 18–20, 43–44, 219–220
Transcendence, 138
Transferences
    ability of psychotic patients to
        form, 128
    age of patient in, 147
Transgenerational transmission,
        43–44
Transitional objects *vs.* transitional
        phenomena, 157
Transitional space, 159–161
Trauma
    centrality of, 77
    hermeneutics of, 82–84

Kohut's understanding of, 187
origin of pathogenesis of, 79–80
pathological accommodation
  and, 223–224
Traumatism, 89
True self, 148, 167, 221–222
  hate and ruthlessness in
    development of, 169
True self–false self, transcending,
  168–169
Trust
  dialogical hermeneutics and,
    43–45
  flexible therapeutic boundaries
    and, 131–135
  hermeneutics of, 31–35, 38–40,
    98–101, 165–167 (*See also*
    Hermeneutics of trust)

U

Überlieferung, 18
Unanalyzable patients
  Ferenczi's work with, 84, 88
  Fromm-Reichmann's work with,
    111–112
  Kohut's treatment of, 187–189
Understanding
  error-proneness of, 194
  in context, 10–11
  interpretation and, 14
  psychoanalysis and, 23
  shared, 25
  work required for, 5–6

Unmediated familiarity, 4
Use of an Object, 143
Useless suffering, 69–70

V

Verbum interius, 35, 40
Verständigung, 17
Verstehen, 17
Vertrautheit, 4
Vicarious trauma, 108
Victim mentality, 67
Vocational commitment, costs of,
  135–136
Voice of the other, 40–43, 61

W

Whole self, 196
Wild analysis, 181
Winnicott, Donald Woods, 7–8, 131,
    220–221
  double hermeneutic of, 168–170
  life and work of, 138–141
  paradoxes of, 143, 156–162
  use of language by, 141–144
Wirkungsgeschichte, 43
Wise baby, 84–88, 231
Wittenberg, Wilhelm, 115
Wittgenstein, Ludwig, 182
Working at the local level, 192, 194,
  199–200
Written *vs.* spoken word, 62

Printed in Great Britain
by Amazon